7 Solutions for Building Your Proactive Chiropractic Practice

7 Solutions for Building Your Proactive Chiropractic Practice

Proven Success Keys to Anticipate and Solve Problems of Design, Growth, and Management

Michael S. Meyer, D.C.

Professional Practice Resources, Inc.
ELKHART, INDIANA

© 2004 Michael S. Meyer, D.C. Printed and bound in the United States of America. All rights reserved. No part of this book may be reproduced or transmitted in any form or by any means, electronic or mechanical, including photocopying, recording, or by an information storage and retrieval system—except by a reviewer who may quote brief passages in a review to be printed in a magazine, newspaper, or on the Web—without permission in writing from the publisher. For information, please contact Professional Practice Resources, Inc., 2609 Greenleaf Boulevard, Elkhart, IN 46514..

Although the author and publisher have made every effort to ensure the accuracy and completeness of information contained in this book, we assume no responsibility for errors, inaccuracies, omissions, or any inconsistency herein. Any slights of people, places, or organizations are unintentional.

First printing 2004

ISBN 0-9744853-4-9
LCCN 2003111436

ATTENTION CORPORATIONS, UNIVERSITIES, COLLEGES, AND PROFESSIONAL ORGANIZATIONS: Quantity discounts are available on bulk purchases of this book for educational, gift purposes, or as premiums for increasing magazine subscriptions or renewals. Special books or book excerpts can also be created to fit specific needs. For information, please contact Professional Practice Resources, Inc., 2609 Greenleaf Boulevard, Elkhart, IN 46514; 574-264-1471.

This book is dedicated to my wife, Carol, who married me when I was a penniless Palmer student and has worked by my side since my first day of practice almost 30 years ago. Many of the policies and procedures in this book are a direct result of her understanding of, and commitment to chiropractic, our patients, and our practice. Without her insights, ideas, and patience, my practice would be mediocre, thousands of patients would never have been adjusted, and this book would never have been written. If chiropractic is truly "Head, Heart, and Hands," she is the "Head" (brains) and I am the "Hands." Together we have the "Heart" to love our patients, our profession, and each other.

Table of Contents

Acknowledgments xi
Preface xiii
Introduction 1

Solution 1
Design Your Office for Success 13

Step 1-1: Location, Location, Location 13
Step 1-2: Effective Layout, Floor Planning, and Decorating 18
Step 1-3: Finding the Equipment That Will Change Lives 23
Step 1-4: Great Forms Result in a Great Practice 26
Step 1-5: Help Your Patients Get the Care They Need
  With an Effective Fee Schedule 27
Step 1-6: Remove the Guesswork With Convenient and Logical Hours 30
Step 1-7: Office Systems—Structuring Your Ideal Practice 32
Step 1-8: Save Lives—Become Known in Your Community 34

Solution 2
Develop a Tremendous Support Team 45

Step 2-1: Preparations of a Successful Employer 45
Step 2-2: Recruiting the Winning Team 49
Step 2-3: Coaching Your Dream Team 57
Step 2-4: Things Aren't Always as They Seem—the "Phantom" CA 59

Solution 3
Devise Systems for Success and Stability 65

Step 3-1: Sharpen Your Message and Focus Your Communication 67

Step 3-2: PI Cards—Eliminate the Paper Chase While Staying on Track   69
Step 3-3: Keep Everyone on the Same Page—Use a Service Slip   73
Step 3-4: Systematize Your Case Management Plan and Appointment Scheduling   75
Step 3-5: Create Specific Procedures for Reappointing Your Current Patients   78
Step 3-6: Develop a Procedure for the Declined Appointment   80
Step 3-7: Manage the Inevitable Missed Appointment   81
Step 3-8: Contacting the Unscheduled Patient   84
Step 3-9: Systematically Recalling the Inactive Patient   85
Step 3-10: Efficient Scheduling and the Appointment Book System   89
Step 3-11: Charting Systems—Accurate and Quick   90

Solution 4
Create Financial Policies to Grow Your Practice ... 97

Step 4-1: Give the Cash Patient Financial Options   99
Step 4-2: Develop Effective Procedures and Reasonable Policies for the Insured Patient   101
Step 4-3: Insurance/Co-Payment Determination for Painless Collections   107
Step 4-4: Play the Third-Party Pay and Personal-Injury Game by Your Rules   110
Step 4-5: Develop Effective and Efficient Insurance Reporting Procedures   116
Step 4-6: Effectively Handling Workers' Compensation   123

Solution 5
Establishing Systems for a Smooth First Visit 133

Step 5-1: Anticipating the New Patient's Concerns   134
Step 5-2: Shaping the New Patient's First Impression   141
Step 5-3: Assembling the Initial New Patient Information   144
Step 5-4: Establishing a Procedure to Verify the Patient's Insurance Coverage   151
Step 5-5: Developing a Strong Doctor-Patient Relationship   152
Step 5-6: Being an Interested, Active Listener—the Consultation   157
Step 5-7 : Letting Them Know That You Know—the Examination   164
Step 5-8: Seeing Is Believing and Understanding— X-Raying the New Patient   172
Step 5-9: Committed and Concerned—Releasing the New Patient   174

◆ Proven Success Keys to Anticipate and Solve Problems of Design, Growth, and Management ◆

    Step 5-10: Successfully Collecting the First Day Fees   176
    Step 5-11: Scheduling the Second Appointment/Spouse at Report   177
    Step 5-12: Committing a Procedural Error—Adjusting on the First Visit   178

Solution 6
Create Lifelong Chiropractic Patients 183

    Step 6-1: Provide Objective—Grade-Based Recommendations   186
    Step 6-2: Making Appropriate Clinical Recommendations   193
    Step 6-3: Building the Relationship—the Case Report   193
    Step 6-4: Making Compliance Easy—
        the Financial Review and Appointment Arrangements   214
    Step 6-5: Manifesting the Clinical Plan—the "Map" Procedure   224

Solution 7
Keep Your Patients Educated,
Excited, and Adjusted 233

    Step 7-1: Renew the Excitement Before
        It Fades—the Reevaluation Procedure   234
    Step 7-2: Help Patients Express Their Excitement—
        Make Wellness a Family Event   243
    Step 7-3: Keep Patients on Track—the Appointment Reminder Procedure   245
    Step 7-4: Maintain Continuity—Forbid Missed Appointments   246
    Step 7-5: "Out of Sight" Must Never Be "Out of Mind"—Patient Recall   251
    Step 7-6: Understand Your Patients—Maintain Control   254
    Step 7-7: Getting a Second Chance—
        Managing Returning Inactive Patients   258

Bonus Solution 1
Generate New Patient Referrals 265

    Bonus Step 1-1: Develop a Referral Atmosphere   266
    Bonus Step 1-2: Consciously Implement Referral Strategies   267
    Bonus Step 1-3: Double Your Referral Sources—
        Spouses at the Case Report   272
    Bonus Step 1-4: Stimulate Referrals from Your Healthcare Classes   273
    Bonus Step 1-5: Explore the Genetic Link—the Well-Adjusted Family   275

Bonus Step 1-6: Make New Patients Happen—
  the Referral Request Procedure 279
Bonus Step 1-7: Remove New Patient Hurdles—
  the Introductory Telephone Consultation 291
Bonus Step 1-8: Stay Alert for the Reluctant Referral 294
Bonus Step 1-9: Turn Inquiries into Patients—
  the Prospective Patient Phone Call 295
Bonus Step 1-10: Ask Subliminally—
  Use Complimentary Consultation and Exam Certificates 299

Bonus Solution 2
Make Success Personal 303

Bonus Step 2-1: Learn to Communicate, Learn to Influence 303
Bonus Step 2-2: Become Overwhelmingly Confident—
  in Your Technique and in Yourself 305
Bonus Step 2-3: Never "Settle"—
  Purposefully Build Your Perfect Practice and Life 305
Bonus Step 2-4: Never "Settle"—Be Happy Where You Are, or Move 306
Bonus Step 2-5: Find a Mentor—Form a "Master-Mind Alliance" 308
Bonus Step 2-6: Never Stop Learning—
  Take Business and Success Seminars 309

Bonus Solution 3
Quantify Your Achievements, Then Celebrate ... 313

Bonus Step 3-1: See the Entire Picture—Statistical Categories 314
Bonus Step 3-2: Running the Numbers—
  Quantitative and Objective Insights 317

A Final Thought 325
About the Author 327
Index 329

Acknowledgments

This book has taken many years to write, and there are numerous people who have provided me with both chiropractic and practice insight and knowledge. But more, friends and coworkers have inspired and coached me along the way. Before I begin, it is only appropriate that I acknowledge the chiropractic giants who I was fortunate enough to call "friends." Dr. Bill Holmberg, and the late Drs. Fred Barge, Cecil Grogan, and John Sayers, Sr., are my "chiropractic heroes." These great men have led and taught me by their words, their actions, and their examples. To this day, I am not alone as a beneficiary of their services to our profession, to Palmer College of Chiropractic, and to every young chiropractor who has followed in their footsteps. Chiropractic and its promise of a better world are, and were, as important to these great chiropractors as life itself. I am lucky to have tipped a glass with each of them.

I must also acknowledge my friends. Dr. Dennis Fitterer, Dr. Gary Street, Dr. Jay Sayers, and Dr. Robert Brooks who allowed me the great honor to serve with them as we led the Palmer International Alumni Association through the turbulent years of the late 1980s and early 1990s. Our laughter, tears, and late night conference calls will never be forgotten.

Everyone needs a mentor. I can only hope my readers are as lucky as I have been to find a friend and mentor like Dr. Gerald Broderick of Elkhart, Indiana. It was Dr. Broderick who gave me my first job, taught me how to adjust patients, and showed me the real meaning of being a chiropractor. From him I learned dedication to my patients and dedication to the work ethic, which is the bedrock of the success I have enjoyed.

Finally, I must acknowledge my friend Dr. Bill Broderick who, through his steady, quiet commitment and love of chiropractic, taught me to understand the dedication that we should all have in serving our patients.

To all these men, thank you for who you are, what you are, and the impact you have had on my personal and professional life.

Preface

Success in every established, and yet to be established, chiropractic practice, is vital to the individual doctor, the future of the chiropractic profession, but more, to the future of humankind. There are simply too few chiropractors and the stakes for humanity are too high. In short, as chiropractors we do not have the luxury to fail in practice or in getting the chiropractic message to the world. The entire human race has an enormous need of our services. The longer I have been in practice, the more I realize that too many of our fellow human beings are mentally and physically ill, or are simply not living life at 100 percent because of the dreadful effects of the Vertebral Subluxation Complex (VSC).

That is why our success is critical, and why we need to produce specific and reproducible step by-step systems, policies, and procedures to ensure our offices will function at the highest levels of service. Just as important, we must develop practices that enhance our lives and produce little or no stress upon ourselves, our staff, and our patients. Only in a stress-free atmosphere can we and our staff function at high levels on a daily basis for long periods of time. Can this be accomplished? Read on.

With every successful practice I have observed, there has been one common thread. Virtually every point of patient interaction—each word, action, form, policy, and procedure—was anticipated, planned, rehearsed, and properly executed. What is more, such procedures were performed exactly the same—every time. There was never any "freelancing," "ad-libbing," or "shooting from the hip" in these offices. In short, these doctors were "proactive" in their approach to their patients and practices.

♦ 7 Solutions for Building Your Proactive Chiropractic Practice ♦

That is what this book will help you do—plan your practice so that you will begin to climb the stairway to chiropractic success. It will give you the seven best solutions (and three bonus solutions) for anticipating and proactively managing practice challenges and for developing a practice that will allow you to enjoy great success by serving both humanity and your own needs. We will help you identify specific points of patient contact that could transition the patient into a lifelong patient or, if handled wrong, discourage the patient from obtaining proper care.

This book is full of specific policies, systems, and words that have been designed, tested, and quantitatively analyzed. They are proven to produce just the right effect on your patients and your practice. Just as your practice problems are seldom individual and separate from one another, these solutions are not sequentially presented. Rather, they will build on a continuum of understanding that can move you forward to grow your practice in a positive and proactive manner. Through these solutions, you will learn how to successfully anticipate and solve specific problems in a positive, efficient, and, of course, ethical manner. This book will help you become one of those successful doctors who know what specific steps to take to make their practice a predictable, profitable, high performance, proactive practice.

Introduction

Dream and Plan Proactively: Lay the Foundation for the Practice of Your Dreams

Are you getting ready to start a new chiropractic practice? Perhaps you have been in practice for many years and are looking for a more rewarding practice. Whatever your situation, your practice must be built on a foundation of personal and professional values, dreams, and expectations.

The challenges that will arise in your practice are always internal and always solvable—as long as that solution is congruent with those same values. Therefore, in any successful chiropractic practice, the real solution to any challenge is always you, the doctor. That is where the successful practice must start. This is where we will begin.

Real success comes from a doctor who is dedicated, confident, competent and ethical in his or her practice and personal life. A life in chiropractic is a "calling," not a profession. Practicing chiropractic is hard work, requiring a strong sense of purpose, mission, and focus. Through the years, other doctors have asked me how to stay motivated and committed. The answer is that nobody can be "on purpose" and focused every minute of every day. But on the whole, the way to be chiropractically strong and confident is to design your life and practice around your personal and professional beliefs and values. To do this in an effective way, you must eliminate any conflict between how you run your practice—and live your life—and the deep-seated personal and chiropractic values and beliefs that you hold.

First, you must begin by deeply examining your chiropractic values and beliefs. Compare those values to your practice, the way you are currently serving your community, and your patients. Be honest with yourself. Think briefly on how you would answer any questions regarding your philosophical commitment to your profession.

Then, take a few minutes to quiet your mind. For a few minutes shut out all extraneous thoughts. Concentrate on simply breathing from your diaphragm and releasing all extraneous thoughts from your mind. Then, ask yourself the hard questions about your practice, your procedures, and your policies in the office. Consider whether or not you are currently practicing in a manner that is 100 percent true to your chiropractic beliefs and values. In short, are you living and fulfilling your purpose every day you are in the office? Examine each aspect of your practice and compare them with your true values in life and chiropractic. Is there harmony or discord? Is there congruency? As you do this exercise, try to eliminate the interference of your educated mind and the temptation to force an answer. Ponder this question for 10 to 20 minutes daily. The answers will ultimately be made apparent. With them, will come the thoughts of your "perfect" practice and the realization of the conflict that is currently resisting your quest to build your perfect, value-based practice.

At the same time, introspectively examine your own life. What is important, really important, in your life? Try to see into your future and develop goals and actions that will make that vision a reality. Your goals and all of the actions that you may take to achieve those goals must be congruent with what you hold dearest, what you value most in life. In other words, each and every goal and accomplishment in your practice and in your life must be based on your personal and professional values. Your successful practice will depend on those people, morals, concepts, and ideals most importance to you, as well as your ability to develop a rewarding and satisfying personal life.

What Do You Value Most?

Before going any further, we must address the important, but often forgotten, law of honoring your personal values. Any achievement attained at the expense of our closely held beliefs and morals, or at the

♦ Introduction ♦

expense of the key people in our lives, will ultimately lead to feelings of emptiness and sadness. To ensure true personal success in attaining your goals, it must be determined that these goals, aspirations, and actions are not in conflict with core personal values.

Simply stated, values involve beliefs, people, concepts, feelings, and morals that are usually formed during early childhood and further developed throughout life. Even when these values are not readily recognized, still they are highly important in building a meaningful and fulfilled life. Therefore, every action, goal, and accomplishment you pursue must be in harmony with your values.

The following exercise will help you determine the values you cherish most in life. Choose 10 from the list and rank them in order of their importance.

- ❏ ____ Achieving personal growth
- ❏ ____ Having peace of mind
- ❏ ____ Having physical security
- ❏ ____ Having financial prosperity
- ❏ ____ Having health and vitality
- ❏ ____ Ability to improve the lives of others
- ❏ ____ Loving and nurturing family relations
- ❏ ____ Having a meaningful job or career
- ❏ ____ Raising happy, well adjusted children
- ❏ ____ Being famous and recognized
- ❏ ____ Being a positive influence in your community
- ❏ ____ Being a positive influence in your profession
- ❏ ____ Having adequate free time
- ❏ ____ Being happy and content
- ❏ ____ Having a close relationship with a higher power
- ❏ ____ Having rich and rewarding friendships
- ❏ ____ Having resources to help others
- ❏ ____ Associating with successful people
- ❏ ____ Having control over one's own destiny
- ❏ ____ Ability to overcome all problems

❑ ____ Living life in a positive manner
❑ ____ Amassing great wealth and possessions
❑ ____ Traveling to exotic places
❑ ____ Having a sense of accomplishment
❑ ____ Being admired as a good person
❑ ____ Having power and influence over others
❑ ____ Having personal and professional integrity

Now, on a separate sheet of paper, create a brief statement embellishing what each of these top five personal values means to you and why they are so important in your life. This list will now form the basis for your goal-setting and decision-making activities. I suggest you keep this list handy, and refer to it to measure every activity and endeavor you involve yourself in both now and in the future. Although your list of values may change throughout your life, you must never sacrifice those that are important to you, unless that sacrifice enhances another value further up the scale.

Once you have discovered what you value most in life, you can begin to develop your plans and actions for building a successful practice and life. Keep in mind that the goals you will be striving toward must never be in conflict with your own personal values. Generating objectives and actions based on what you truly value will ensure that when you do achieve your goals, they will not be empty or meaningless. Every year or so, as you revisit and update them, your values will change along with your life circumstances. Some values will become less important—some more important.

"How Vivid Is Your Dream?"

We all aspire toward a brighter future, but without a dream, there is nothing but shadowy, indistinct, and fleeting thoughts as to what you might want your future to be. Right now, being in practice or continuing to create your ideal practice may only be a dream. However, you must dream carefully and succinctly. As a chiropractor, the dream that will ultimately become your practice is extremely consequential, because your practice will ultimately become the vehicle that will allow you to realize most of your other dreams.

♦ Introduction ♦

Next I would like to encourage you to take a few minutes (or a few days) and create (or recall) the vision of what your "dream practice" will one day be. Only this time, see it clearly and more distinct than you did earlier. Make notes in a spiral-bound journal or notebook. As you do, use each of your senses. See the walls, the floor, the colors, the furniture, your adjusting tables, and of course—the people. In your mind's eye, look at everything. Hear what is going on. What are you saying to your patients? What are your patients and staff talking about? Is there laughter…children's voices…music? Use all of your senses. Do you want to see lots of senior citizens? If so, can you smell the little old ladies' perfume? Try to dream of the practice that you would build if you had no limitations of time, money, talent, self-confidence, energy, and support. Then, write down every concrete detail that you see, hear, smell, and feel. High intention in dreaming of the perfect future practice is the starting point in bringing that dream to reality.

Most importantly, you must reduce every aspect of your dream to writing. Writing it down on paper makes your dream tangible and real. It will keep you focused and on track. Writing down your dreams will give them substance and make your visions real. Take the time and make the effort to see and then to write down every detail of your perfect practice. Then, we will begin building it.

Dreaming of Your Perfect Practice

For those readers who are trying to decide on where to locate after college, or who are considering a change, it is important to chose the right area to practice, the right staff, the right patients, the proper procedures, and every other single detail of your practice. Describe the attributes you visualized in your practice. For example, if you are trying to visualize the place where you will you will ultimately live, establish your practice, and raise your family, try to imagine the attributes of the region (e.g., warm climate, cold, Midwest, mountainous, lakes for fishing, trails for hiking, culture of a big city, shopping, etc.).

Go ahead, visualize and describe the type and location of your ultimate, ideal office (e.g., big city, rural, professional building, free-standing building):

Describe the look and feel of the internal environment of your office.

_____

_____

Describe your staff in as much detail as possible. What are they wearing, doing, saying, etc.?

_____

_____

Describe the age, gender, etc. of the typical patient that you want to see.

_____

_____

How are your patients taking care of their finances? Are they making new appointments as they leave?

_____

_____

What is your average income generated by the services you render to your patients and your community?

_____

_____

What type of cases do you want to see and what percentage of your practice do they comprise (e.g., wellness patients, subluxation only, pediatrics, personal injury, athletes, all types, etc.)?

_____

_____

Can you see yourself in this "dream practice" yet? Can you see yourself adjusting patients? Quickly? Efficiently? Effectively?

◆ Introduction ◆

Will you practice straight subluxation-based chiropractic or will you utilize modalities and therapies? If so, what and how often? On whom?

_____

_____

What is your technique? How good are you?

_____

_____

What are your patients saying (are they complaining, happy, appreciative, sick, healthy, etc.)?

_____

_____

What are you discussing with your patients (chiropractic, health, the weather, the ball game)?

_____

_____

What do your patients and your staff want and expect from you, both professionally and as a person?

_____

_____

Will you accept insurance, personal injury cases, cash practice only, a combination? Describe:

_____

_____

What other attributes of your "dream practice" have you envisioned? Describe them in as great a detail as possible:

_____

_____

What is the major contribution that you would like your practice to make to society?

_____

_____

What will others in your community say about you, your practice, and chiropractic?

_____

_____

What overall impact will your practice have on the lives of the people in your community?

_____

_____

Obviously, the only right answers are the answers that are right for you. Once you have answered these questions, you must begin to acquire the necessary knowledge to develop the practice you have outlined. By attending seminars or associating with established doctors who have already figured out how to make your type of practice successful, you will gain the knowledge to build your own.

While the choices are yours, I suggest you consider developing a practice that will (at least initially) bring all types of patients into your office. This way, you may address your patients' initial condition-based complaints. While doing so, you will have the opportunity to hone your adjusting and patient management skills. And you will enhance their health and lives by converting them into well-educated chiropractic patients who have chosen a healthy subluxation-free lifestyle. While such a patient and practice transformation will require a lot of effort in the application of specific educational procedures and management policies, it is certain that developing patients who understand the intrinsic the value of chiropractic, will bring about a stable, highly rewarding practice.

Remember too, most of the patients who enter chiropractic offices are well steeped in the allopathic paradigm of healthcare and the treat-

◆ Introduction ◆

ment of named diseases. Consistent, well conceived, and effectively implemented patient education can, however, bring about understanding and acceptance of the chiropractic model of healthcare. Strategies for developing and implementing such a plan will be addressed later in this book.

As you begin to see your practice, you can now start to formulate actual goals and take the steps necessary to realize just such a practice. Your practice will be a special and unique entity. Through your commitment to your values and the building of your perfect practice, you will serve your fellow human beings. That great service will enable you to realize your personal and professional dreams. But, as a final warning, as you begin to develop this wonderful practice, never forget to balance every choice, every commitment, every action, and every decision you make against your list of personal values.

James C. Collins and Jerry I. Porras, authors of *Built to Last: Successful Habits of Visionary Companies,* contend that "core values are an organization's essential and enduring tenets—they are a small set of general guiding principles; not to be confused with specific operational practices; not to be compromised for financial gain or short-term expediency." Whether you are just beginning your practice or if you have been at it for a while, start with your core values. If necessary first take the time to identify your personal and chiropractic values, see your vision, set your goals, and then have at it.

The Big Difference

People are often divided into the "haves" and the "have-nots" of the world. There are the successful and the unsuccessful, the happy and the unhappy. Quite often, the biggest difference between such polar opposites is that one group establishes a system of values, envisions a desired future state, and then sets specific goals—both long- and short-term—to realize that vision. The other group simply does not. The other group wanders through each day of their lives tending to the survival needs of the moment. In doing so, they never get much past worrying about their survival.

Among those who understand their core value system, who dream and set goals, the rate of success is infinitely greater. Another huge difference is that one group writes down their goals and visions; the less successful group does not. Norman Vincent Peale has said: "Only three percent of the people on earth ever commit their values, desires and ambitions to writing, but they accomplish more than the other 97 percent put together." Of course, we all dream of certain achievements in our lives. Unfortunately, most of our dreams never get beyond the dreaming stage because they never become actual concrete, physical objects. Most exist as fleeting glimpses in the inner recesses of our minds bouncing back and forth between unconsciousness and a transitory wish. Begin now to give your dreams a physical existence. Cement them in writing as clearly and as boldly as you can. Place them in a conspicuous spot and look at them frequently.

When you finally understand your core values, embrace your dreams, and set your goals, you may then develop a mental image of a possible desired future for your practice. With such an image, you can plan and carry out the actions necessary to help you realize your dreams. The rest of this book does just that—it provides the information and insights needed to help you build your practice and use it as a vehicle to help you to realize your professional and personal dreams. The ideas in this book are meant to serve as both a map and a service manual to take you on a wonderful journey through life as a successful chiropractor. They will help you to build your practice, serve your community, and thereby enjoy the love, respect, abundance, and happiness you deserve. The suggestions contained in this book can help you understand your values, realize your dreams, and accomplish your goals. Implementing these strategies will enable you to achieve the life and practice that you want and are worthy of—by successfully serving humanity.

Key Points

- Any achievement attained at the expense of closely held beliefs and morals or at the expense of people in your life will ultimately lead to feelings of emptiness and sadness. To ensure true personal success in attaining your goals, it must be determined that these goals, aspirations, and actions are not in conflict with core personal values.

- Keep in mind that the goals toward which you will be striving must never be in conflict with your own personal values.

- The dream that will become your practice is important because your practice will ultimately become the vehicle that will allow you to realize most of your other dreams.

- Take the time and make the effort to see and write down the details of your perfect practice.

- When you understand your values, embrace your dreams, and set your goals, you may then plan and carry out the actions necessary to help you realize your dreams.

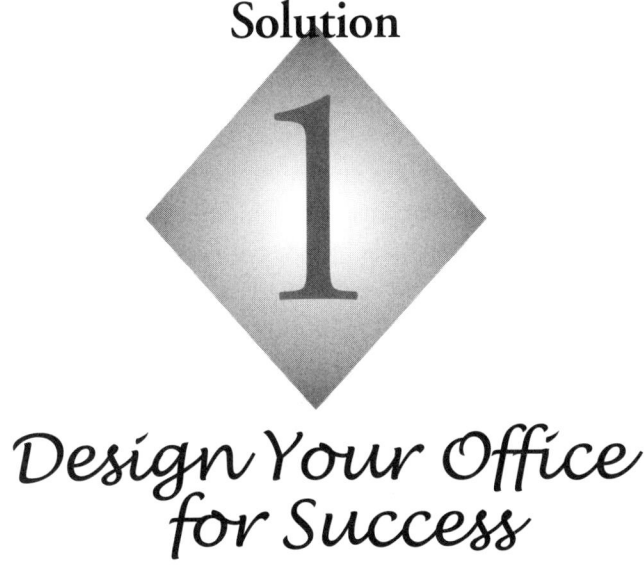

Solution 1

Design Your Office for Success

Establishing your new practice or evaluating your current practice is the most important business activity you will do. Opening your office correctly will heavily impact the success of your practice and your life. If you are currently in practice in an established office, you should use this section to help you to evaluate your current office. If you are opening a new office or just starting practice, Solution 1 will serve as a guide to the successful establishment of a great office.

Step 1-1: Location, Location, Location

When considering setting up a new chiropractic practice, or even the success of an established practice, nothing is as important as office location. Much early time and effort must be placed on selecting just the right location.

The best way to find a new location or to properly assess an existing one is to obtain a large map of the community from the city, county, or state planning office. This map will give great detail of the area in which you currently practice or are contemplating opening your new office. With this map, you will begin your demographic study of the area. The first step (with the aid of the Yellow Pages) is to mark the locations of all of the other chiropractic offices, medical clinics, hospitals, health food stores, and other health professionals in the community. This will give you a general idea of the distribution of the other chiropractors, physical therapists, walk-in clinics, etc. Then, scout out these establishments and the immediate community. Try to determine any impact the location of each may have on their apparent success or lack of success.

Next, identify the locations of the major employers, retail areas, and residential areas. The local chamber of commerce will have needed statistics for this task. Then, identify the major north-south and east-west thoroughfares connecting the community and most importantly the major employers with the major residential areas. If possible, try to visualize the commuting and traffic patterns of the community and mark them with a highlighter on your map.

And finally (possibly most importantly), consider contacting the construction supervisor of the local utility companies (telephone, gas, and electric) and inquire as to the projected areas of new service construction. Future growth of most modern communities is planned well into the future. Knowing the planned future construction of the infrastructure in a community will give insight as to growth, long before the first stores, homes, or factories are built. This knowledge may help impact your decision of where to locate your office within the community.

While you should not be too concerned with opening up in the same neighborhood as other established practices, this exercise will show you areas of underserved populations that may be a likely location for an office. The average new doctor, without the above knowledge, may jump at any opportunity to locate in these areas, only to realize that it was a mistake later. Please remember though, if you consider locating in neighborhoods that appear to be underserved, it is critical that you check out these areas carefully. The questions you should ask yourself are: "Why is this area underserved?" "Does someone know something about the community and the area that I don't?" "Why have other doctors avoided this area?"

Answers to these and similar concerns may be easily answered by discussing them with local businesses, realtors, and the chamber of commerce. This exercise of identifying prospective locations actually may show you what areas you may want to avoid as much as where you may want to consider, thus avoiding the mortal mistake of locating in the wrong area of town.

Next, with the help of city or county planning or even the utility companies, you should be able to identify areas of projected community growth as well as the type of growth. Whenever you can, determine if an area you are interested in is convenient to patients. (Again, is it near or between major employers, shopping centers, and residential areas?) The ease with which you will fill your practice with new patients—and ultimately, lifelong patients—depends to a great extent on convenience, visibility, and accessibility.

Early and long-term success depends heavily on your office location. Therefore, you must carefully study the demographics and psycho-graphics of potential patients in the area you choose, and compare them with the patients you described in previous exercises. No matter how much you like this location, the main question you must ask yourself is "Do my dream patients actually exist in this area?" If not, it will obviously be difficult to build the practice of your dreams without having the type of patients you wish to care for.

A well-traveled street that is readily recognized and is in an area with economic growth potential is a great place for an office. High visibility is also important. Be sure that once the office is established, both the building and the sign are visible and recognizable from the street. Also, it is important that your office and sign project the type of image you want to portray to your patient and community.

Office location, visibility, accessibility, recognizability, traffic flow, and image portrayal are critical to practice growth. The only type of marketing more important and more effective than the office where the practice is ultimately located will be the doctor's own personal promotion of him- or herself and the practice. Be visible. Be convenient. Be accessible.

Another extremely important consideration is that the prospective office must have good access to and from the street. It should have close and ample parking, and be handicap accessible from the parking lot to the office door. Remember, you will be caring for patients who are elderly or possibly immobilized. Not only must they be able to get from their cars to the front door, they must also be able to enter and exit the parking lot with as little stress as possible. Therefore, avoid busy intersections where patients may have difficulty entering or exiting safely. Look at the traffic flow into and out of the parking lot. How difficult would it be if you were elderly or handicapped? Your practice is going to grow and that, from time to time, you will get behind schedule. If there is not adequate parking space, the lot may become congested. Nothing will frustrate patients more than for them to arrive for their appointment on time then not be able to find a space to park, thus making them late for their appointment.

Also, whether setting up in a metropolitan area, the suburbs, or out in the country, always try to find a location where patients have direct and close access from surrounding communities. Is the location near an interstate or a community-linking highway? Are there exits near the location from surrounding highways? Are the exits marked and recognizable? Often, it helps patients to find your office (or even to choose to come to your office) if they are familiar with or can easily identify the specific area or neighborhood. Even better, you might try to find a location near a well-known landmark, store, or intersection. Familiarity with the surrounding area is often an important factor in prospective new patients' choosing your practice.

If you wish to house your practice in its own freestanding building, or even if you are sharing a building with others, don't settle for anything that is not professional on the exterior or the interior. Choose a location that presents a professional image of you and your practice. Avoid anything that may appear seedy or run-down or in a questionable part of town.

Obviously, signage is critical. Your sign should be professionally designed and constructed, visible, readable, and beckoning. As a 24-hour advertisement for you and your practice, you should never cut costs on your sign. A good sign is an investment that will pay for itself many times over. Be sure it is visible from all directions and lit at night. Use dark or bright colors for the background of your sign with white or light, contrasting lettering. This will make your sign stand out from its surrounding background. White or light signs tend to blend in and become unnoticed, even with dark lettering.

Before committing yourself to signing a lease or buying a building, always check with local (city and county) municipalities about zoning laws, especially how they may restrict site usage and signage. Don't take for granted that just because a sign may already be in place that it is in accordance with local zoning laws. Check it out with the city and county zoning board before making any commitment to purchase or lease a specific property.

Both the office and its sign will serve as important marketing tools. They will be symbolic of the doctor, the practice, and the profession day in and day out, for years to come. Choose both carefully.

Another consideration is whether or not the site has potential for physical expansion of the office as the practice grows. Having to move to another office just after getting established is both costly and hard work. Instead, try to plan for your ultimate success. Plan for growth. Look for a location where the site allows for room to increase your floor space if necessary. If you are locating in a strip mall or leasing a building with other tenants, ask the landlord for a "first right of refusal" on adjacent floor space when it becomes available. Such a concession should always be put in your lease. If you are building new, or building out a leased space, try to floor-plan so that any future expansion might be accomplished with minimal disruption to the original floor plan and so that there is continuity to your practice while construction is being completed. Again, do not overlook the availability for adequate parking for both the increased patient load and the increased staff down the road.

A concept that usually addresses all of the above considerations is to locate in a neighborhood strip mall or "out lot" with a large grocery store anchor. These facilities typically satisfy all the needs for location and accessibility and often leave room for expansion into adjoining units. An important aspect of locating in or near strip malls is that someone else has already (professionally) done the all-important traffic flow analysis and demographic surveys. The criteria used to locate these types of projects are close to those mentioned earlier, and will fill your needs. In addition, your office will be located somewhere where your patients and potential patients usually go on a regular basis. Just make certain that your rented space is highly visible from the street and your sign is prominent. Being hidden in the side or back of such a complex quickly defeats the purpose.

Obviously, you should expect to pay a premium price for the prime location, but the benefits will quickly outweigh the costs. Here you can usually start with a minimum square footage and acquire more as your practice grows. Again, be sure to include in your lease agreement a "first right of refusal" to adjoining units whenever they may come available after you begin to outgrow your initial space.

Step 1-2: Effective Layout, Floor Planning, and Decorating

In designing any office, a few basic considerations must be addressed. While your planned technique will dictate much of how your floor plan will be configured, special attention should be given to several other factors. Whether you wish to practice in an open environment or in individual adjusting rooms, every office must have certain basics.

Front Desk/Reception Area

Every office must have a front desk and reception area. Openness of the front desk area is critical for the office to convey friendliness and a sense of the practice and its staff being open, available, and service oriented. However, there must also be some concessions made for privacy in the collection of fees and making of future appointments. If the front desk is separated from the entrance and the reception area by a wall, that wall should have a large open window so that the front desk chiropractic assistant (CA) can see and welcome every patient as they enter the office. In addition, the front desk should be situated so that the CA will have full view of the reception room, the entrance, and the main hall where the patient activity is taking place.

Another important consideration is that the front desk area has adequate desk or counter space. In a modern office there must be room for a computer, telephone, small copier, typewriter, appointment book, and any other tools the CA will need to do a good job. When setting up the front desk area, be sure that the telephone is within easy reach of the appointment book or the computer terminal. Planning for telephone jacks throughout the office is important, but nowhere is it more important than at the front desk. Mounting the phone on the wall (within easy reach) can make it handy, freeing the desk space for other items.

Shelving and filing areas also should be within easy reach of the assistant. If you plan on using the patient information card system (discussed later), try to locate the storage trays close by. In a perfect office, the CA should never have to leave the desk area to retrieve or file cards or patient files. He or she should be as close as possible to the primary work station.

Also, the front desk should have a second raised countertop for the patients to sign-in as they enter and on which to write their checks as they leave. This front counter should be approximately chest high (40 inches) so that the patients do not have to bend over after their chiropractic adjustments. It should also be high enough and wide enough so as to serve as a visual block for the actual working level of the CA. For your front desk to be compliant with the Health Insurance Portability and Accountability Act (HIPAA), patients must not be allowed to see the appointment book, computer screen, day sheet, patient records, or other confidential matters that may be on the front desk. Simple strategic planning of the construction of the front desk will effectively protect patient privacy.

While supply storage need not be at the front desk, close and adequate storage for all business supplies that may be needed by the CA during the course of the day is important. Again, all efforts should be made to design the front desk area so the CA never has to leave the area to perform the job.

Reception room layout and location is also critical for your convenience and that of your staff and patients. The reception room should be in close proximity to the most frequently used rooms in the office. Most often, these are the adjusting rooms. Carefully planning for both the patients', staff's, and doctor's movements through the office can eliminate wasted time and effort, which might otherwise be a bottleneck and limit your practice growth. By reducing the amount of walking both you and the patient will have to do, office efficiency will be increased proportionally.

Depending on the size of the waiting area, the practice, and the doctor's ability to stay on schedule, a minimum of four to six good chairs are needed in the waiting area. If large families are an element of the practice, more will be required. When choosing chairs for the reception area, consider that very often patients will be symptomatic and in pain. Appropriate seating should not only offer good support, but should also be easy to get into and out of. Sturdy reception room seating should include firm upright chairs with arms that assist the patient's use of this furniture. Consider the large and obese patients who will surely be members of your practice. Choose chairs wide enough to accommodate these patients as well.

The projection of warmth in the reception room is also important to help put the patient at ease. Besides the liberal use of items that project an attitude of health and life (such as an aquarium or vibrant plants), using warm tones of paint will project an area of friendliness and warmth, putting anxious and overwrought patients at ease. In offices that are lit with harsh fluorescent lighting, the addition of incandescent lamps or track lighting will actually soften the bright whiteness of the fluorescent lighting.

Remember that patients are bombarded daily with media stories, announcements, advertisements, and news reports of subjects that may be the opposite of the chiropractic message you are trying to instill in your patients. Therefore, you must always pay close attention to the reading materials provided throughout the office. Magazines should be carefully screened for anti-chiropractic messages or pro-allopathic slants; apologies should never be made for obvious censorship in your office. Whenever possible, substitute good chiropractic literature.

Adjusting Rooms

The next areas of the office to consider are the adjusting rooms. The adjusting rooms should be in close proximity to the front desk and the reception room. If you are using multiple rooms, the doors should be as close as possible. The proximity and ease of flow between each room and the front desk will influence your ability to limit your steps and ultimately the miles traveled throughout your career. To the extent that patient transport and your movements throughout the office are limited, the office will be more efficient.

In a typical chiropractic practice, two adjusting rooms are usually ideal, but if floor-planned properly one will be just as, if not more, efficient. For most types of techniques, two rooms will allow you to be adjusting a patient in one room while the CA is preparing and placing the next patient in the other. This way, you may move from one room to the next without waiting for patients to proceed from the waiting area to the adjusting room. If you are efficient and can move quickly between patients and rooms, it may be necessary to have three adjusting rooms so that the CA can actually keep up with you and the patient flow.

If, however, the reception room or patient holding area is set up properly, and is in close proximity to the adjusting area, one adjusting room may be sufficient. If the office has a separate holding area for patients who are right outside the adjusting room door, the patient may be sent to this area, and then the doctor may take them into the adjusting room as the previous patient leaves. Remember that in any practice setup, patient flow, efficiency, and speed are critical for the practice to grow.

In the adjusting room itself, you must also strive for efficiency and energy conservation. This can best be accomplished by never moving the patient from one piece of equipment to another unless absolutely necessary. Whenever possible, you should develop a technique that allows the patient to be adjusted on only one adjusting table. Also, to facilitate note taking, it may be helpful to have a countertop on which to write patient progress notes. Make sure it is installed at a level that lets you write the necessary notes while standing up. Sitting down, writing notes, then getting up with each patient is time-consuming, leads to extraneous conversation and fatigue, and is never time efficient. The adjusting room should also have wall hooks on which patients may hang their jackets and sweaters. Otherwise, patients will lay their articles of clothing on the adjusting equipment, desk, or wherever it seems logical to them. Invariably, however, these articles will be in your way.

If possible, always try to have windows in the adjusting rooms that open to the outside. An open window will freshen an adjusting room faster than any mechanical ventilation system or chemical air freshener.

Examination/X-Ray/Consultation Room

The examination/consultation room is another important consideration. In tight quarters, this room may double as an adjusting room, but it is better to have it separate. In many instances, the CA may be reviewing appointment scheduling or financial agreements in this room, and to tie up an adjusting room for other purposes may slow you down. Better yet, combine the examination, consultation, case reviews, and the x-ray into one room. In the processing of new patients, it is far easier to do everything in the same room and not have to move a patient (gowned or otherwise) to different rooms during the course of the first visit.

In the examination/consultation/x-ray room, all the equipment needed to complete the first visit should be present. A consultation table with four chairs, an examination table, and all of the miscellaneous tools to perform a good examination should be included in this room. If the consultation/examination area is not in the x-ray room, it should, at least, be in as close proximity to the consultation/examination room as possible. Since this room will be the least used room during the course of the day, place it farthest from the front desk area. This combination room will not only serve as the new patient induction room, but should also be the site for the ensuing case report. Here, x-ray view boxes, charts, chiropractic exhibits, and other needed items for delivering the case report will be kept as well. It is also recommended that no background music be piped into this room. Such background noise is often distracting to both you and your patient during the consultation, it may limit your ability to hear vital sounds during the examination, and it will be distracting to both doctor and patient during the case report.

Whatever room ultimately houses your x-ray machine, its setup is an essential consideration in your initial office configuration. Here is where you will spend a huge chunk of your startup capital. Once you have found your office and decided which room will house your x-ray equipment, ask your x-ray dealer to assist you in planning this room and the darkroom. I have found that any salesperson who is truly interested in selling a machine will be more than happy to tour your prospective facility and recommend the setup of your x-ray/examination suite. Such assistance may also be an indicator of future service after the sale and should be a major consideration in selecting equipment and distributors.

Doctor's Private Office

Another floor-plan consideration is your private office. This area is where many doctors unnecessarily devote too much floor space and spend too much of their startup funds in purchasing desks, bookshelves, and seating. Many set up beautiful private offices, anticipating impressing patients during the initial consultation, only to find they are the only one to see the room. The private office should be your workroom rather than a place to impress patients. The patients will be much better served if you invest more in a good table and set of chairs for the consultation area (where the patients will be anyway). Your private office should not be used as a consultation room. In the course of the day, you may be engaged in many other projects, from writing reports to figuring payroll. The private office is a place for you to go to perform these tasks without having to clear your desk before each new patient is brought back.

Patient Education Center

Finally, a key consideration in setting up your office for success is the development and placement of a Patient Education Center. This area may be set up in any room, but the consultation/examination room may very easily contain the patient education center as well. This is the area where all case reviews and progress reports will be delivered. Therefore, it is important that it be outfitted with view boxes, charts, and, if utilized, a VCR or DVD player and television monitor.

This area should contain a corner countertop where you and your patients can sit knee-to-knee to discuss the patient's case and provide chiropractic enlightenment. There should be chairs for patients and their spouses. Position them so that the occupants can see the countertop, wall charts, TV monitor, and view boxes.

It is also recommended that the doctor's chair in this room be a swivel-type secretarial chair. Such a chair takes up less room and allows you the freedom to swivel between charts, view boxes, and written materials as you present the patient's case report.

Remember that an effective, highly functional, and successful practice can only grow from a well-designed, well-functioning physical plant. You must give enormous consideration to your floor plan as it dictates patient flow and doctor efficiency, and will encourage or limit your success in establishing the type of practice you desire. Your floor planning will encourage and determine both practice growth and the character of your practice.

Step 1-3: Finding the Equipment That Will Change Lives

Most chiropractors I know have a special relationship with their equipment. Many even give loving names to their hi-lo tables. You will serve your patients every day for many years on your adjusting table and you will rely on your x-ray machine for the insight to make proper decisions in the care of your patients. Securing the necessary equipment involves major choices that must be made in setting up the new practice or updating an existing one. Of course, the needed equipment is going to be dependent upon the technique you will be using. But the less money you spend in opening your practice, the sooner you will be profitable. Use discretion, but at the same time do not spend your money on junky or used equipment simply because it is cheap.

The old cliché is true—you get what you pay for. This advice is especially true when purchasing x-ray equipment. Be especially particularly wary of buying used x-ray equipment. If you are purchasing used equipment, always buy from a reputable dealer who will both install it and guarantee it for at least a limited time. Also, when possible, you should check with the previous owner. Ask why he or she discarded it, if the equipment was easy to use, if it routinely took good pictures, or if it had any known problems. Ask how hard it was used. The same advice also applies to x-ray cassettes and screens, as well as used processors. Usually the doctors you will speak to have traded their old equipment for new, and will not have a vested interest in your purchasing it. You should get straight answers.

Often, new doctors must decide whether to lease or purchase the equipment they need to open their office. This decision depends on the lease arrangements, and will be one of the early questions for your accountant. Fundamental pros and cons do exist. Leasing may allow the new doctor to begin practice with new or better quality equipment. Sometimes, with leasing you may have little or no initial capital outlay. Without spending your meager startup capital on equipment, you may preserve your money to be used for working capital during the first few months after opening. Remember, however, that leasing does come with monthly payments and sometimes steep interest rates.

Also remember that any equipment that is leased does not become an element of your net worth. Purchasing your equipment outright results in no ongoing payment commitments (unless funds were borrowed to purchase the equipment outright). In most cases, interest rates on borrowed money are often more reasonable than for leases, and the equipment can be depreciated by you, not the leasing company. Again, the major argument against outright purchase of your equipment is that it may drain initial operating capital, leaving little left to pay rent, payroll, or utilities until the patient load has been built and a steady stream of income is established.

While I counsel each client and you, the reader, to seek the wisdom of a good accountant who is familiar with you and your situation, a good rule of thumb often promoted by most accountants is that the new doctor lease big-ticket items and purchase smaller items. Alternatively, for more established doctors it may be of greater benefit to utilize a tax deduction or to depreciate owned equipment. Again, many different considerations and situations exist that would sway a new doctor between leasing equipment and buying. Of special concern in choosing to lease your equipment is whether to opt for one with a buy-out provision at the end of the lease. In the end, the decision should always be made with in-depth counsel from a trusted accountant.

After finding a location and deciding on the floor plan of the new office, your attention should now turn to finding and securing professional supplies and office equipment to run the office. The best way to find out what companies are providing the best and most reliable service is to ask other area doctors who their suppliers are and where they purchase their equipment, office forms, x-ray supplies, etc. State conventions are a good place to meet area suppliers and service companies. Even if you do not attend the convention itself, you should visit the convention display areas, introduce yourself, and become known to the exhibitors. Suppliers and distributors will soon be knocking on your door eager to serve your needs. When they do, welcome them warmly and treat them with professional respect. They may soon become a wealth of information and support.

In terms of equipment, many of the higher quality tables are often not actually assembled until the order has been placed. Therefore, it is important that doctors who plan to open a new office after graduation ascertain the actual delivery times on the equipment that will be purchased. Such lead-time considerations will be a major factor in developing a timeline for opening the practice. Since it would be rather difficult to open an office without an adjusting table or other critical equipment, contacting equipment distributors long before graduation to determine the needed lead-time is a good idea.

Step 1-4: Great Forms Result in a Great Practice

Effective forms and business supplies are the vital track on which your practice will run. They will set the tone for your patients, and insure compliance of office procedures and policies by your staff. Great forms will also keep the doctor on track clinically.

A professionally prepared, comprehensive, and well-understood system of patient forms must be in place before the first new patient ever walks into the office. Prior to purchasing or developing such a system, you must anticipate every action and interaction that will occur with each and every new and established patient. From that anticipation should flow a well-conceived procedure that will quickly and efficiently gather the patient's personal, clinical, and financial information into a system of forms that are interwoven and sensibly integrated in the management of that case.

From the beginning, a basic patient account-keeping system is needed. The original pegboard system sold by many business supply companies is tried and proven effective and efficient. The startup costs for a computer-based system will be significantly greater in the beginning, but such costs will quickly even out when the expense of purchasing yearly pegboard receipts and other associated forms is considered.

Business cards are another consideration needed for getting the new doctor's name and other important information out to the community. Business cards help to build the practice in many ways, but you do not have to spend a great deal of money on them to be effective. Many of the business supply catalogs will custom print professionally designed cards at a reasonable cost compared to local commercial printers.

Another important consideration is whether or not to computerize your office from the beginning. Today, with the lower prices of both computers and software, a computer is the logical way to go. Many doctors already have personal computers, so it seems only reasonable to decide on an inexpensive software package and become familiar with it before opening the doors to the new practice.

Today, many software programs also have computerized scheduling available. Being packaged with basic patient and practice management programs, this software makes managing a practice easier and faster than in earlier days. Remember that both you and your front desk staff must be proficient and comfortable with the computer software before installing the patient files, financials, and the appointment book and doing away with the hard copy systems that may have previously been in place. The wise approach to incorporating a new system may be to run a dual system with a pegboard and receipts, and to keep an actual appointment book until all of the glitches have been worked out of the new system. Keep in mind that just one mistake—a failure to backup or a software snag—can paralyze an office for months.

Step 1-5: Help Your Patients Get the Care They Need With an Effective Fee Schedule

The bedrock of all successful financial dealings with the patient, and the ultimate success of the practice, is the establishment of a fair, honest, and effective fee schedule. To ensure the success of setting your fee schedule, keep in mind that it must be reasonable, logical, and in line with other similar practices in your community. In addition, the schedule must be simple—simple enough that it may be easily communicated in a concise, understandable manner to all patients and prospective patients who may inquire. A fee schedule should never be a barrier to practice growth; instead, it should be seen as affordable and reasonable to the average patient you wish to attract.

Being at either end of the spectrum is unwise and never productive. Being the cheapest will give the appearance of a doctor who does not provide high quality care and will attract the type of patients who may not fit into your concept of a "dream" patient. Being the most expensive will exclude many patients needing care and limit your new patient flow. Very high fees may also result in low patient visit averages (PVAs) or lead to high accounts receivable and collection problems. Therefore, never set your fee schedule at the level of the cheapest in town nor with the most expensive.

The best way to establish your fee schedule is to take a survey of fees the other doctors in the area charge. Call other offices in your area and the surrounding areas and inquire as to the cost of a first visit, with x-ray, initial exam, etc. Inquire about regular visit charges and what their payment policies may be. Then, align your fees with those already successful offices. The successful practices have figured out what the majority of patients in the area can afford for good care. Their various fees are usually at a level that appears professional yet not overpriced.

Once the parameters of your basic fees are established, actually sitting down to design a fee schedule that supports the type of practice you wish to build can be a real challenge. Again, you should go back to the initial questions that you answered as to what your "dream practice" actually looks like. Visualizing your ideal patient, you can then work out a schedule that will attract and retain this type of patient.

Do you want a family practice? Then you must design a system that will allow entire families to afford to come to your practice. Do you want a wellness practice? Then your fee schedule and collection policies should reward patients for getting checked and adjusted on a regular—asymptomatic basis. Do you want a "condition-based" practice? Then your fee schedule and policies must allow patients to afford frequent initial care. If your "dream practice" is to be filled with "dream patients," you must tailor your fee schedule to the type of patients you wish to fill it with.

Above all else, remember that the fee schedule is only a small component of building your proactive practice. In the end, it is the actual financial policies that are developed and put into place that will dictate whether patients can afford your care, rather than the fees you charge. Properly designed and presented, each and every policy, procedure, and script should compliment and enhance the practice's fee schedule and should encourage the type of patients and the type of practice you desire.

Whether you want your practice to be all cash, insurance-based, or a combination of the two is another consideration. If you decide to establish a cash-only policy, you must remember that your fees must be kept affordable. Patients and prospective patients have only a specific number of dollars that they can and will spend for nonemergency healthcare. In a "cash" practice, educating and repositioning the patient will increase the value of the services being rendered and therefore predispose the patient to make a greater investment in his or her health. Therefore, in a cash practice especially, you must have your own personal philosophy, communication skills, and patient education well developed and designed before any fee schedule will work well.

An "insurance" practice comes with another important set of considerations. While keeping your fees in the same range that is usual and customary in your area, you must still charge enough to offset the cost of extra staff and doctor time. Remember that inherent with an insurance practice is the additional time spent by doctor and staff in completing paperwork, processing forms, and the costs associated with electronic billing. Also to be considered is the accumulative cost of lost interest incurred over the years by waiting for a delayed payment to be made, or the amount of services that simply may become uncollectible.

My suggestion is that you design a fee system that handles both insurance and cash patients. Doctors who wish to have only a cash practice will eliminate a large number of patients who prefer or even must use their insurance benefits in order to receive care. By developing such a system, you will allow "condition-based" patients to enter your practice utilizing the benefits of their insurance plans, then with the help of your patient education and communication skills as they transition from condition-based into wellness, you may also convert them into cash-paying patients. Properly designed, your fee schedule, policies, procedures, and scripts will allow patients to come to your practice as either "cash" or "insurance" patients and then, to stay for a lifetime. Of course, by itself, a fee schedule will not build the perfect practice. But it is an important element of an overall system of procedures and policies that will allow your dream practice to develop. Overpriced, underpriced, or simply ill-conceived, a fee schedule can be a huge factor in preventing the development of your proactive practice.

Later in this book, we will discuss the actual policies and procedures needed to properly implement your fee system. However, at this point, you should begin to consider what the actual charges for the services you will render would be. Survey your colleagues, consider the type of patient you wish to attract, and frame a vision of the type of patient you will consistently care for. Then consider the development and setting of your fees.

The practice of chiropractic is a critical service to humanity and the world, and your fees should be established in a way that encourages the people in your world to receive the care they need. I have always felt that if I were going to collect $1,000 per day, "I would rather see 50 patients for $20 than 20 patients for $50." Yes, as doctors of chiropractic we have assumed a mission and, as B. J. Palmer called it, "a sacred trust." Please do not allow your fees to interfere with that mission or to destroy that trust. I encourage you to make your fortune through service to the multitudes rather than collecting large fees from the few.

Step 1-6: Remove the Guesswork With Convenient and Logical Hours

Establishing office hours in a new community (or changing hours in an existing practice) is an important decision that can have a far-reaching impact on the growth and stability of your practice. In establishing your office hours, the two most important considerations are that your hours must be convenient for the people of your community and simple for them to remember. When the patient needs to make an appointment or to call for one, they should be able to easily remember when the office is open and the phones are answered. I have found that office hours can only be memorable if they are consistent from day to day. Office hours that vary from one day to the next may seem to be more flexible for patients, but if too varied, they may be confusing and frustrating instead.

Most importantly, when designing your schedule, make certain your office hours are compatible with the schedules of the patients you wish to attract to your practice. If you wish to attract families, your hours should be extended into the evenings when the children are out of school and Mom and Dad are off work. If you wish to care for factory workers, your hours should be designed around the shift changes of the local factories. To be most effective, your office hours must make you available to patients (and to prospective patients) at times when those patients can most easily make appointments and come to the office without disrupting their regular work, school, and daily routines.

Adjusting office hours to those of area employers is a good way to know that your practice is going to be available when patients can come. You can best determine your office hours in two ways: first, call the personnel office of neighboring employers and ask about hours and shift changes for the majority of their employees. Second, determine the hours of the other doctors, not just the chiropractors, in the area. Try to figure out why they have set their hours. You may also try to be open during the hours they may not be serving the community, making you available for emergencies or new patients.

Keep in mind that new patients are priceless to a new practice. Not only are new patients a source of needed income to meet early practice overhead, but they also represent the apex of a referral pyramid that may bring an ever-increasing number of new patients into the practice for years to come. Therefore, each new patient is absolutely critical to your success. For this reason, the new or growing practice must be open for extended hours during the first few years. It may represent a sacrifice of personal, leisure, or family time during those early years, but for the success of a new or expanding practice, you absolutely *must* be available when both established and new patients call. The difference between failure and astounding success of your practice may be just a few new patients and the resulting referral pyramids that are obtained simply by being available when other doctors are not.

Besides the establishment of a well-conceived schedule of hours, you must discipline yourself to physically be in the office for all established hours. The idea that it is slow in the office or that the last patient is gone at 4:30, so "let's go home" is dangerous to your confidence and that of the staff and the patients. Such lack of self-discipline will ultimately affect the growth and stability of your practice. If you have posted office hours, you must discipline yourself and your staff to be there every minute of every posted hour.

There is one exception to this rule. In this day and age of beepers and cell phones, it is possible for you to leave the office to meet people and promote the practice within the community. While self-promotion and other community awareness activities are a good use of downtime, the office must always have a CA on the premises, the doors open, and the lights on. In the case of a walk-in patient or an emergency, you must be responsive and close enough to be able to return to the office within a very short period of time. You should never leave the office during office hours unless a staff person is there to handle calls that come in, any patients who stop by, and the many and varied other situations that may arise.

Remember, the two main considerations for setting office hours for a new practice are to schedule hours that are convenient for the majority of people in your community, and to have somewhat extended hours in the early morning, evening, or weekends, making you available as much as possible.

Step 1-7: Office Systems— Structuring Your Ideal Practice

The establishment of efficient office systems from the very first day the practice is open will not only increase the odds for early success, but will allow for growth and a smooth transition to the large practice in the future. Such systems are described in detail in the remainder of this manual. Implement these ideas as quickly as possible. Remember, they have been developed by years of trial and error in large, busy practices. They not only encourage initial growth in new practices, but provide efficiency in large established practices.

One of the most important systems that should be instituted with the first patient of a new practice is the "patient information (PI) card." The patient information card is a bi-folded card that contains virtually all of the information you will need to care for the patient on all subsequent office visits during the lifetime of that patient. It does not replace having a full-sized folder on each patient; the folder is needed to store correspondence, case worksheets, third party payer information, and other items that must be kept on hand. The patient information card does, however, prevent the pulling and filing of entire folders on each visit. It greatly increases the efficiency of the front desk, and the ease with which you may review, record, and track patients.

Included on the patient information card is a brief synopsis of the patient's initial consultation, an annual calendar for posting multiple appointments, a box for recording and updating diagnoses, a section for listings and objective findings, and a large area devoted to entering patient comments and adjusting procedures. The front of the card should contain all of the patient's personal, and, if needed, third-party information. Besides the thoroughness of the basic information contained on the patient information card, layout and organization is extremely important. In development of the patient information card, special attention to the actual layout of the various panels reduces appointment time, streamlines note taking, and immeasurably improves doctor productivity.

Another system for growth and efficiency in a chiropractic practice (especially a practice that does not use physical therapy or other procedures preparatory to the adjustment) is the concept of the clipboard and numbered room system. This is a system based on the concept that the patient is usually smart enough to find their way to a specifically numbered adjusting room and then return to the front desk without being escorted by a staff member. This system is extremely efficient because it allows patients to move themselves through the office with minimal staff involvement, saving the practice both time and money. In most cases, the clipboard and numbered room system speeds up the office visit process by removing the banter that usually occurs in the hallway between the patients and the staff member escorting the patient to the room.

To implement this system, you need only to number the adjusting rooms in a logical manner and then have correspondingly numbered clipboards and plastic holders on the walls where the patient will place their clipboard. On the patient's first regular visit (usually the third visit) to the office, the CA will escort the patient to the adjusting room and show them how the rooms are numbered. They will then show the patient where to place the clipboard with the chart and where to sit in the adjusting room while they wait for the doctor. On all subsequent visits, the CA will attach the patient information card to the clipboard and give it to the patient, and instruct the patient to go to the proper adjusting room and have a seat. With this procedure, the CA need never leave the front desk or provide any further assistance. After the adjustment, the doctor can simply complete the notes and comments on the patient information card, mark the day's charges on the service slip, record a time interval for the patient to return, and then send the patient and chart back to the front desk for exit processing.

Another means of effectiveness and efficiency is for the practice to have well-designed and written statements of financial policies for new patients. Written policies and patient agreements will speed the patient indoctrination process and bring the patient into compliance with the office's set policies quickly with little divergence from the established policies. When you are developing written policies for the patients, remember to keep them brief and easy to read. Try to write at a seventh- or eighth-grade level to ensure comprehension by all patients.

Efficient and quick adjusting techniques will also set the stage for growth. Try to set a specific structure for each visit. By doing the same procedures in the same order on every visit, the patient will become comfortable, knowing what to expect, and you will then finding yourself practicing with much more efficiency and much less stress. Remember that the patient is in your practice to have their subluxations adjusted and their health returned or maintained—nothing else. Get them in, give them your chiropractic best, be specific in your adjusting, and let them go.

A coded diagnostic system comprised of all the ICDA codes normally used in your practice speeds up the process of providing insurance diagnosis and diagnostic updates. By designing an alphanumeric code meaningful to you and your practice, you may eliminate searching for the proper code, and then having to write the full code. This code may then be recorded on the patient information card so that all departments will have access to it when needed. Once a code is established, most computer software systems will allow that coding to be implemented in the program for later retrieval of that specific diagnosis onto billing statements and insurance forms.

As stated earlier, a well-conceived system of office forms for attaining patient information, clinical processing, financial management, and third-party reporting will endow the practice with procedures that are simple, effective, and fast. Try to simplify and combine multiple forms to reduce the paper shuffle in your office wherever possible. Simplicity combined with comprehensiveness in each department is essential for a smoothly running practice.

Step 1-8: Save Lives—Become Known in Your Community

Becoming and staying known (established) in the community is the first and most important consideration in building a new practice and in maintaining the momentum of an existing practice. It is the easiest and preeminent way for those who are subluxated, sick, and suffering to find you. You owe it to your community, yes, even to all of humankind to get out into your community and become known.

Following are a few ideas on how to become known, liked, and accepted by neighbors and prospective patients. First, it is extremely important that you become involved in your community. Community involvement, such as joining civic groups, the chamber of commerce, volunteer organizations, and church groups will produce the opportunity for you to meet many of the influential members of the community. It should be remembered that to become involved in these groups and activities solely for the purpose of getting new patients will quickly become apparent and such efforts will backfire. Community involvement must be for the right reasons. As a professional member of your community, it is the right thing for you to do—it cannot be merely for personal gain. Community involvement and service lead to community awareness, respect, and appreciation. It is this same respect and community recognition that will ultimately help fill the new practice, or help keep an established practice full. Such activities are much like planting a garden. The planted seed will, in time, bring a bountiful harvest.

One of the first things many people do when they move into a new community is to visit and ultimately join a place of worship. With each church, synagogue, or mosque you visit, you must be sure to make yourself known to the pastor, rabbi, or other leaders. Later, when you select a place of worship, don't just attend. Get involved by being the first to volunteer to help. Serve on committees and be available when needed. Arrive early and be the last one to leave after services are over. In short—serve, but serve for the right reasons. As you do, you will meet people who will appreciate you, admire you, become patients, and recommend others.

Intramural sports (YMCA, park, or church leagues) are another good way to become involved and known in your community. Participate as a coach or sponsor. Always conduct yourself in a professional manner, even in the heat of competition. Your community is watching and forming opinions about you—not just as a participant, but as a person and a professional.

Civic groups are another way to become actively involved. Before joining any service club, however, I recommend you personally visit all of them in your community. Try to find one that is a good fit with your values, ideals, and personality. Look for a club that has the greatest number of members who suit your personality and with whom, ultimately, you would like to fill your practice. Visiting and joining a service club is a good way to become known to others who are involved in your community. Once you join, become active. Ask to be placed on the fellowship committee or other highly visible committees. But, do not expect new patients immediately. Most people will not come to you until you are known and accepted.

The local chamber of commerce is also a good way to meet many important and influential members of your community. Before actually joining the chamber, however, sit down with the director and discuss the organization. Find out how you might best serve the community and the chamber and ask to immediately be placed on any committee(s) that interests you before you agree to join.

One of the obvious ways to meet people and make friends is by interacting with your neighbors. You must be both friendly and visible in your own neighborhood. Spend time outside of your home, especially in your front yard. Be a good neighbor. Take care of your own yard and take care of it well. Play with your children in your front yard. Wave at passersby and make an effort to meet your neighbors. A quick way to meet your neighbors is to contact your local police department and enlist their help in organizing a neighborhood watch group. You may also consider hosting the initial meeting at your house and personally go door-to-door, introducing yourself and inviting your neighbors to the meeting.

In short, the best way to become established and known in your community is to meet new people. The more people you know, or who know you, the faster your practice will grow and the more successful it will become. Set a goal to meet three new people every day. How you can meet and make an impression is limited only by your imagination. But you must meet others, and you must make a good impression. Never be shy or afraid to greet and talk to others.

Public speaking is also a great way to become known and to attract new patients. While you do not always have to make presentations about chiropractic, you should always make sure that your audiences know who you are and what you do. In accepting any speaking invitation, the selection of audiences is key. Be sure to develop topics and select audiences based on the type of patient (your "dream patient") you wish to attract to your practice and then speak about them and their interests and concerns.

Public speaking allows you to develop and then present topical seminars with information that focuses on problems or concerns consistent with the type of prospective patient you wish to fill your ideal practice with. For instance, if you wish to attract working men and women to your practice, you might develop programs dealing with safe work habits, lifting, bending, stooping, etc. If you wish to attract children and young families, you might develop and present programs about mothering, child development, and so on. Be sure you sound sensible and confident in your message and ability.

Also, in an effort to become known in your community, you should develop quality brochures and other products to identify yourself and your practice. Make sure that everything you use is consistent with your desired image. High-quality business cards, letterhead, and brochures all make an important impression on prospective patients. Also remember a negative effect can just as easily be elicited if these items are of lesser quality and reflect poorly on your professionalism. The brochure should include your biography, office hours, directions to the office, your credentials, philosophy of practice, appointment policies, unique features of doctor or facilities, etc.

Another effective consideration for getting your message out is to produce an audio brochure of your practice. How many times in the past few years have you had a patient, friend, or someone "out of the blue" ask you to listen to an audiocassette tape about the newest multilevel marketed health panacea product? If you have, at some point you may have asked yourself why every multilevel company in the world has gone to this form of media to get their message out. Okay, maybe you haven't. But if you did, the answer is simple: It works and it is cost-effective. Remember, these companies employ marketing geniuses to get their message out and to get people to buy. They research and test-market. They know what works and what does not work. Their research tells them that audiocassettes get listened to.

If you think about it...almost everybody these days has a cassette or compact disc player in his or her car, and just about everybody drives his or her car—every day. Voilà. A captive audience. And, listening to a tape or CD is easy. People don't have to take time out of their busy day to listen. They don't even have to take their eyes off the road. They just insert a tape or CD into the player and are entertained while they go to work, the store, or to pick up the kids.

This could be a tremendous marketing/educational tool for your practice as well. I suggest you consider producing your own audio brochure(s) for your practice. It is inexpensive, doesn't take much time, and, when done in your own voice, it makes you an instant expert and a known personality to the listener.

But first, you need to decide what your message will be. Do you want to educate your new patient about chiropractic before their case report? Do you want to ask for referrals, or to introduce a prospective patient to your practice? Maybe you are aiming for a combination of all of the above. In fact, you may have several messages and therefore the need for more than one recording. Once you decide on your message, sit down with your office brochure and all of the other brochures and patient education materials that are either decorating your office walls or blowing around your parking lot. Cull out the "big ideas" and the information you want your patients to know about you, your practice, and the philosophy, art, and science of our profession. Then, arrange it into a logical sequence and wordsmith it into an informative script. Make your script conversational and your voice a combination of enthusiasm tempered with warmth. Be careful not be too long or too detailed. In fact, the briefer you can make it, the better. Most around-town car trips last three to five minutes and we want our listeners to get the whole message in one listening.

Once you have your message scripted, sit down with your cassette recorder in a quiet room and begin recording your message. Remember to speak slowly and distinctly. Make at least three recordings, listening to each with an objective ear. Listen to your intonation and your emphasis on certain topics. Practice a few times, then give the recording to a family or trusted friend to listen to and evaluate. Tell them that even though it may hurt that you want their honest opinion. Then, a day or two later, cut the final version.

If the quality from your recording is not acceptable, you might try a local recording studio (found under "Recording Services" in the Yellow Pages). These services usually charge by the hour for you to go in and make your recording. They will give you high quality sound and professional "bump" music before and after your message. They can even supply a professional voice to introduce you if you wish.

From the master, you can copy the final product on your own equipment at home. Or, you may have the recording service reproduce it for you. The costs are usually quite affordable. A full service printer or graphic artist can easily create labels for the tapes and "J" covers for the cassette case, which will give a professional look to the whole project. If you have it professionally done, you might even consider having your photograph put on the cover so your listeners can visualize the person they are listening to.

Take a tip from the marketing "pros." Make your own five-minute recording to get your messages out. Your patients will love it and it will provide multiple benefits to your community and your practice as it is passed from one person to the next.

Newsletters do get your name out into the community, but often they are expensive, time-consuming to develop, and do not have the hoped-for results. If you decide to produce a monthly newsletter, you can mail or give your newsletters to patients, attorneys, barbershops, grocery stores, health food stores, etc.—anywhere people gather. I recommend, however, that you be sure to measure their effectiveness and the return on your time and money invested. Using a special offering with a coupon that must be returned with the desired action will enable you to track its effectiveness. Only by quantifying your response can you determine the effectiveness of a newsletter, mailing, or advertising.

A good way to encourage a person that expresses interest in your services to take action and come into the office is to give them a complimentary consultation and examination certificate. This is simply a small certificate (about the size of a dollar bill) that you can present to someone who may be a prospective patient. This certificate will extend to that person a complimentary consultation and examination.

To be most effective and to move the patient to action, the certificate should have an expiration date of less than two weeks on it. This dating will produce a sense of urgency and increase follow-through.

People love to be appreciated. Saying "thank you" to everyone you can think of is a great way of making a good impression and being remembered. Sending personalized thank-you notes is an easy, yet effective way to show your appreciation to those who, during the course of your day, should be acknowledged. Make an effort to send at least three thank-you notes every day. Send them to every person you can think of who does anything for you, your practice, or your community. These small gestures of appreciation can be both fun and extremely rewarding in the goodwill they foster.

When opening the new office or practice, remember to utilize the business announcement section in the local newspapers. Write up an announcement as you would like it printed and supply a resume and a black-and-white photo. Always supply more text than you know will be used. It will frequently be edited to some extent. At the same time, place an opening announcement or advertisement in the same local papers. Ask that the running of the paid advertisement coincide with the article in the business announcements section (on the same page, if possible). Then, don't forget to send a thank-you note to the editor of the paper, in appreciation for the exposure.

Another good way to become known in your community is to become a certified CPR and First Aid instructor by the American Red Cross. Once you are fully certified, you can offer your services to teach first aid and CPR to local industry and community organizations. While this activity is not necessarily chiropractic-oriented, it does present you as knowledgeable, in charge, and someone to be respected and sought out when a chiropractic need does arise.

While a listing in the local telephone Yellow Pages is a must for survival, you must make sure to determine which phone book is the most popular book in area. If you are going to place a display ad, it should be just large enough to get the information you want displayed. In today's Yellow Page market, it is difficult to determine which book is the most widely used, and the competition is fierce and expensive. The general rule for Yellow Page advertising is that "if you can't pay...don't play." If you are going to rely on a Yellow Page advertisement for new patients, you must remember that the larger the city, the larger the ad should be. But, if you are actively promoting yourself, and your office fits the parameters described above, the need for a large ad or any at all is much less. To be cost-effective, you may use a **bold** listing so people can find you when they are looking for you, but a display add may be a waste of money that could be used elsewhere much more effectively.

Another option, if you cannot afford to match the largest ad in the telephone book, is to place a bold listing and a one-to-two-inch "in-column" ad. An in-column ad is not only less expensive, but it is listed in alphabetical order. So there is a double advantage if your name or practice listing falls early in the alphabet.

Before placing a display ad, make certain the sales representative clearly and honestly explains the company's policy on ad placement. In most instances, the ad is placed by size first and then by seniority in that size category. Be sure to always review the current issue of the phone book(s) in which you intend to advertise. Given that others in your category will not change the size of their ads, you will get a good idea as to the placement of your display advertisement, again taking into consideration size and seniority.

The main features of a Yellow Pages advertisement should include a description of the location of the office, especially noting any nearby landmarks or cross streets, your hours, and phone number in large bold type, and the statement, "New Patients Welcome." If you have a good logo that reproduces well, use it prominently. It is seldom conducive to developing a high-quality practice to advertise the "treatment" of various conditions unless your ideal practice consists of specializing in certain conditions. Advertising specific conditions will almost certainly attract patients who are seeking care for the specific condition listed, but may actually cause others to rule out your practice if their problem is not among your list of complaints. Unfortunately, this tactic may actually limit prospective patients who are searching for an office from the telephone book. The patients who may be attracted may also be symptom-relief oriented, and therefore, may or may not fit into the type of practice you are striving to build. In my experience, practices that advertise symptoms or conditions often find that it results in lower patient visit averages.

Also, advertising specific clinical techniques or anything else the average person will not understand may actually be a waste of valuable ad space. Don't use red, unless it is an integral element of your logo. Red is often subliminally interpreted as being aggressive, confrontational, or just plain irritating. In short, if you decide to place a Yellow Page display ad, be classy: Advertise benefits not gimmicks. Do not cheapen yourself or your profession by advertising any free service; it is unnecessary, unprofessional, and sounds desperate.

As soon as you determine a place of practice, call the telephone company and the Yellow Pages and ensure your listing in the next phone book issued. Even if you do not have an office, but know the general area, you need to have a phone number reserved for you that will guarantee a listing in the next issue. This may cost a few dollars initially, but is a good investment when compared to not being listed in the telephone book for your entire first year.

If you do invest in a display ad, be sure to track the number of new patients generated by the Yellow Pages, and especially which book they used to find you. This tracking will help you to make educated decisions for future advertising. I also recommend you track the type of patients who enter your office because of a response to a Yellow Page advertisement. If you are going to spend thousands of dollars each year for a Yellow Page advertisement, you should at least make certain you are attracting the kind of patients with whom you want to fill your practice.

Another consideration is that if you choose to call your practice anything other than your own name, pick a name that falls early in the alphabet for in-column listings. Check out other listings in your category and determine where your listing will be placed.

Finally, beware of Yellow Pages sales representatives. They are well trained, often pushy, and usually effective at convincing an inexperienced customer to buy larger ad space than needed. Know what you want before speaking with them, determine your budget, and then stick with it. Do have at least a bold, in-column listing in both the white and Yellow Pages.

Key Points

- When considering the establishment of a new chiropractic practice, or the success of an established practice, nothing is as important as location.
- You must give enormous consideration to your floor plan as it dictates patient flow, doctor efficiency, and will encourage or limit your success in establishing the type of practice you desire.
- Remember, the less money you spend in opening your practice, the sooner you will be profitable in practice.
- Becoming and staying known (established) in the community is the first and most important consideration in building a new practice and in maintaining the momentum of an existing practice.

Solution

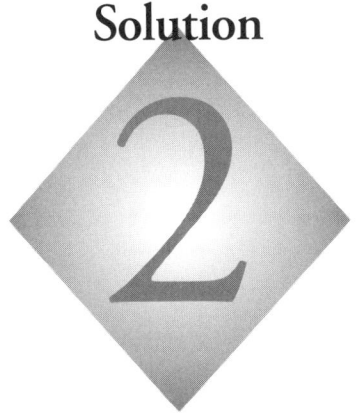

Develop a Tremendous Support Team

Developing a strong and effective support staff is the most important, and at the same time, most difficult managerial undertaking you can do to insure a vital growing practice filled with satisfied patients. To accomplish this feat, a great deal of preparation is needed before you tackle the hiring process. Job descriptions, an operations manual, and an employee handbook should all be written and in place before the first "help wanted" advertisement is placed or the first person hired.

Step 2-1: Preparations of a Successful Employer

The Job Description

The first step in developing a new practice staff or improving an existing staff is the development of comprehensive and in-depth job descriptions for every position in the office. Job descriptions are important for several reasons. They provide order and delineate positional functions and responsibilities for the performance of all vital activities in a systematic and organized fashion. In addition, job descriptions are perfect tools for bringing a new staff person into the practice. Job descriptions are vital in helping new employees understand the position they are assuming. They orient the new employee into the practice and define the working relationship of each position with the rest of the staff. The job description also addresses the scope of decision making that the employee will have in performing these job functions. It should address the degree of communication with other employees and patients and the scope of such communications. The job description should also include a statement that allows you to assign other duties and responsibilities to the employee.

The complete job description will include four different elements. The first step in writing a job description is to determine the actual functions that must be performed by the person filling that position, and assign a title to the position. Once that has been determined, a brief summary of the position, generally describing its purpose and functions as it relates to the other positions within the staff and the overall attainment of the practice's mission, must be developed.

The third component of the document will list the qualifications, the educational background, and any experience that the eligible applicant must possess to be considered for the position described. Included in this section should be a description of the ideal personality attributes and skills that the successful candidate must possess to function successfully in the position.

The main body of the job description should be a point-by-point listing and explanation of each of the responsibilities of the employee. In writing this portion, always remember that the job description is simply a listing of all the functions to be performed in the particular position being described. It is not the "how to" or an explanation of the procedures required in performing these functions. Such directions will be addressed in the operations manual that will be discussed later.

The job description is a valuable tool in selecting prospective employees. By clearly delineating duties to be performed and identifying the actual skills needed to succeed in the position described, the employer can better match the attributes, skills, and experience of applicants. By accurately spelling out the degree of skills and personal attributes needed, the job description can also be used to provide objective assistance in determining various pay structures for the different positions in the office.

◆ Develop a Tremendous Support Team ◆

The Operations Manual

The next personnel management tool whose development is a must for every successful practice is the operations manual. Here, you should spend a lot of time and energy to adequately describe, in exact detail, each procedure that needs to be performed and every situation handled for the office to function properly. You must also describe exactly how each department or position will interface with others in the accomplishment of all given tasks. Essentially, the manual will reduce to writing the specific, detailed application of all of the procedures that must occur for each position fin the office to run efficiently and effectively. And it should summarize the expected standards and benchmarks that are used to measure the degree of success of all tasks to be performed.

As you develop your operations manual, try to include each and every position in the office, every function to be performed, and then give specific step-by-step instructions as to how to accomplish that. Your operations manual will be complete only when it provides the written procedures and solutions to every situation and every task that may occur in the day-to-day operations of the practice.

If you already have employees, the development of the operations manual can be made much easier and implemented more successfully by enlisting the help of your current employees in its development. Ask your employees to keep a list of everything they do on a daily, weekly, and monthly basis. Then, they should write out, step-by-step, how they perform each task. At that point, you can either correct and rewrite the procedure as necessary, or simply leave it unchanged and make it an element of your standard procedures as described in the operations manual. If you enlist the help of your staff, be prepared for an eye-opening experience. You will find that many tasks are being completed that you are not aware of or that they are being performed in a manner totally unlike the manner in which you wish them to be completed. Remember to compare the list generated by your staff with the list contained in your job descriptions. Typically, there are many functions being performed that are not included in the job description.

Once this incredible task is completed, the practice will begin to take the shape, structure, and order of the ideal practice that you desire.

In short, the operations manual is a document that essentially takes every single function described in the job description and says "this is how we do it here." It is the office's official "how-to-do-it" guide. It designates the steps that (without modification) must be taken to successfully perform each activity described in the job descriptions. Like the job descriptions, the document must be simply written and easy to understand. Use words with no more than three syllables, avoid professional jargon, and keep sentences short.

Finally, even if your staff is motivated, well trained, and experienced in their positions, variations and mutations of procedures will naturally occur over time. Good management dictates that you create an operations manual, and then observe and correct any variances that may develop. An operations manual is a "living" document where updates, revisions, and better ways of doing things should be recorded and made policy when they become apparent. I recommend that whenever you observe a staff person deviating from procedure that, before you dictatorially correct the action, you discuss with that person the reasons he or she has deviated from posted procedure. You may find the person has actually figured out a more efficient or effective way of performing a particular task. If so, you must then decide if it warrants replacing the original procedure. If it does, you should update the operations manual to reflect the new procedure. If so, do not forget to congratulate—even reward—the employee. If not, you should review with the employee the reasons for doing the task as directed and reinforce adherence to proper procedure.

The Employee Handbook

Effective employee management dictates that you not only describe the job and train the employee on how to perform the duties of the position, but you must present basic policies, expectations, and consequences for the employee prior to the establishment of the employer-employee relationship. The advancement, discussion of, and acceptance by the employee of policies and expectations will set the tone and produce the framework necessary for the successful development of a long and mutually satisfying relationship between the employee and the practice.

The employee handbook is the employer's tool for establishing the rules, employment policies, and guidelines for dress and employee behavior. Not only will a handbook establish these guidelines, but it will also outline the consequences of not adhering to the practice rules as stipulated in the manual. In addition, the employee handbook should describe all of the benefits that are provided to the employees of the practice.

Basic contents of the handbook should include an introduction welcoming the new employee to the practice. It should also include a listing and general description of all employment policies, such as vacations, time off, sick leave, personal leave, pregnancy leave, family care, insurance, etc. In addition, it will spell out the structure for performance reviews, disciplinary procedures, safety policies, policy for determining raises, holidays, codes of dress and behavior, and any other policy or provision where agreement should be reached between the employer and the employee prior to hiring the employee. The whole idea behind the employee handbook is to address and reach an agreement with the employee on any expectation, question, or employment situation that may arise.

Two other important topics contained in an employee handbook are an employment-at-will clause and a sexual harassment statement. An employment-at-will clause addresses the fact that the employee has not been hired for a specific length of time but will serve until either party wishes to discontinue the relationship. In other words, this clause specifies no guaranteed length of employment. The sexual harassment clause should simply state that no form of sexual harassment would be tolerated in the office and spells out the actions to be taken should such a situation occur.

Finally, there must be a clause giving the employer the right to revise any aspect of the handbook should circumstances change, or new ones arise. Remember, presenting the handbook to a new employee embodies an agreement between the employer and the employee. The employer says, "This is what we expect, and this is what we offer." The employee says, "Okay, I agree to work for you under these terms." When unilaterally changing a mutual agreement, care should be taken to explain the necessity for the change and to make it fair to both parties.

Step 2-2: Recruiting the Winning Team

Recruiting the winning team for your practice is one of the most significant duties you will have in all of your professional life. Unfortunately, just like raising a child, a lot of it is "made up as you go along."

This is true at least for the first few children as well as employees. And, like children, employees never come equipped with an owner's manual to answer the important questions that will certainly arise.

After being an employer for almost 30 years, I think the importance of getting the right staff person(s) ranks right up there with choosing the right spouse. Not only must your employees be efficient and effective in their jobs, but you will also spend an inordinate amount of time working closely with these people. Those you hire should not be a reflected image of you as the doctor and employer. However, it is important they hold similar values, ethics, and morals.

The recruiting and hiring of staff can generally be divided into three categories: advertising the position and accepting resumes, interviewing and testing, and hiring and integrating.

The most effective vehicle to get the word out about an available position open in your practice is to list it in the classified section of the local newspaper. Listing the same notice under every appropriate classification will bring in a broader range of prospective applicants. To attract the most serious and qualified people, include the job title, a brief description of the duties, and basic skills and attributes that the applicant should possess. Be careful, however, that you do not indicate a preference based on the sex of the applicant or use any language referring to age.

If you wish not to identify the practice in the newspaper, you may ask that resumes be sent to a post office box. Better, however, is to ask the prospective applicants to drop off a resume or to fill out an employment application at the office.

Whenever an application is made in person, do not actually interview the applicant at that time. It is better to wait and interview several applicants at a convenient time. The reason for this is twofold: first, the applicant may not be prepared or have the time for an interview and may not present themselves as well as possible; and second, by interviewing several applicants consecutively, the interviewer will get a comparative assessment of each in relation to the group. Also, accepting applications in person, allows you (or a trusted staff member) to assess the person's appearance, mannerisms, professionalism, and interactions with staff and others (strangers) prior to offering them an interview.

It is often beneficial to have the staff member accepting the application, rate the applicant on a scale of one to five or just offer basic observations about the applicant. You can ask your staff to make any notes appropriate about the applicant's personality, appearance, and interactions when the resume is dropped off. Be sure this is done on a separate piece of paper that can later be disposed of, not on the resume or the application. Such a procedure will often allow the employer to weed out persons who may not be appropriate for the position before having to spend time interviewing them. In addition, asking another established employee for input into the process and listening to his or her suggestions gives the established employee a personal interest in ensuring that a recommended new employee succeeds.

If the applicant has a resume prepared, you may accept it at that time, and when they return for an interview, give them your own employment application to complete. Although generic applications may be purchased at the office supply store, it is important that yours contain the necessary information exclusive to the practice. In addition to the usual name, address, and social security number, your application should ask about any criminal convictions (other than traffic violations). Hiring someone who has a criminal record and giving them access to patient files may result in charges of negligent hiring practicing against your practice should patients or their privacy be violated in anyway by this person. The application should also ask for a description of the type of employment the applicant desires, what hours and days he or she would be available to work, and the applicant's minimum salary requirements.

Your application should request a listing of the applicant's educational accomplishments, major areas of study, and any special activities or awards. But most important is the applicant's recent history of employment. Obtaining a chronological list of former employers, positions, duties, starting and ending salaries, and reasons for leaving each position will give you a good idea as to how long the applicant has held previous jobs and his or her long-term dependability.

Ask for at least three references, two of which are familiar with the applicant's work habits and abilities. Beware if at least one of the references does not come from the list of previous employers. The listing of references should then be followed by a signed release, asking permission to contact the references and permission to investigate all statements made in the application. At the end of the application include a statement certifying that all information given is true and accurate with a place for a signature.

The Initial Interview

Once all applications and resumes have been received, appoint a staff member to arrange interviews with those who appear to be suited for the position. Interviews are best scheduled over lunch or at the end of the day for the convenience of both the applicant and the practice. The initial interview is a time to assess the applicant's personality, poise, and communication abilities. The interview should be conducted in a friendly nonthreatening environment. From the onset, the interviewer should make an attempt to put the applicants at ease and to gain their trust.

Questions should be open-ended in nature, not answered with a "yes" or a "no," so the applicant has an opportunity to speak at some length. Technically, it is illegal for an interviewer to ask anything personal that is not strictly job-related. Therefore, always avoid direct questions that will lead the applicant to disclose their age, marital status, number of children, nation of origin, or sexual preference. Health or disability questions should be avoided, as well as questions pertaining to religion. It is possible to develop open-ended and general questions that lead the applicant to disclose information about which you cannot ask.

Probing statements such as "Tell me about yourself" or "Tell me about the jobs that you have had in the past (duties, responsibilities, what you liked and did not like)" or "What was the hardest aspect about your last job?" will provide useful information. These open-ended leading questions invariably will give the interviewer more information than can be legally or tactfully asked.

The interviewer should also be taking note of the applicant's poise, communication skills, ability to think quickly, apparent levels of stress, and personal mannerisms that may qualify or disqualify them for the position offered.

As soon as the interviewer obtains a good appraisal of the applicant, the initial interview may be concluded. Explain to the applicant that there are several other interviews to be conducted over the next few days, and those among the final two or three applicants will be called back for a final interview and testing. At this point, remember that the interviewer does not accept questions from the applicant beyond giving them a brief explanation of the duties of the job. The interviewer should never say anything that may be interpreted as a promise of employment or even that the interviewee *will* be called back for a second interview.

Checking References

Once all the interviews are completed, you and the other staff members who met the applicants should meet and review each application and discuss their personal appraisals of the individuals. Quite often, the personality presented to the interviewer will be quite different from that presented to other staff members. You will find it amazing how different the initial impression of the applicant will be between the interviewer and the other staff who have interacted with the applicant. After such discussions, select the top two or three candidates and begin to check references. Reference investigation in a professional office is critical. Checking references will substantiate the applicant's claims of experience and competence, leading to an informed decision on hiring the best person. As mentioned earlier, in certain situations, failure to investigate references could actually expose the employer to legal liability because of negligent hiring.

In investigating the references and job history, employment dates, job titles, attendance, and rates of pay should always be confirmed. In addition, specific questions on industriousness, conscientiousness, and ability to work and interact with others are not unusual. You should also ask open-ended questions of the previous employer to gather helpful information that may have otherwise gone unknown. By simply asking whether the previous employer would rehire the applicant or if there is any other pertinent information, you may gain valuable insight that could influence your hiring of the applicant. In some cases, the cooperation by the person named as a reference may not be totally forthcoming. To help avoid this situation, the employer may consider getting a signed statement from the applicant, authorizing the former employer to supply the requested information. This release can then be faxed to the former employer with a cover letter stating that all information will be kept confidential, and may include a list of specific job-related questions that may be asked prior to the actual inquiry.

The Second Interview

After determining the top two or three candidates and checking references, the time arrives for the final interviews. It is usually best for you (or the person doing the final interview) to make the phone call advising the applicant that he or she is among the few being considered for the position. This gives the caller the opportunity to judge the applicant's telephone voice and professionalism. The applicant should then be invited to participate in a second interview and a basic skills test. In doing so, the caller should be warm and enthusiastic but, again, never imply that a position will be offered.

Before the second interview is conducted, the applicant should be asked to complete a brief skills test, just to make certain he or she actually possesses the ability to perform the job functions. Such a testing procedure should always examine the abilities and skills dictated by the job description.

As with the initial interview, the interviewer should ask open-ended questions, again looking for poise, confidence, and quick-thinking abilities. These questions, however, should be more in-depth and pointed, requiring evidence of abilities to perform the job requirements. Asking the applicants to describe their strengths and weaknesses in such a job setting, as well as their preferences or dislikes on various subjects in a similar employment setting, will quickly differentiate the better applicant.

The most important ingredient of the decision-making process is going to be based on the employer's ability to systematically and objectively rate the applicants and to effectively distinguish the most promising applicant from the others. Such a system requires the identification of the five most important attributes required to fill the position.

Reviewing the job description for the position may easily identify these attributes. These five attributes should then be weighted by giving a possible five points for the most important and one for the least important. Immediately, after the interview, the interviewer should rate the applicant in each category. The final score (the total of all categories) compared to the other applicants, will then give an effective and objective basis for decision making.

It cannot be emphasized enough that hiring people who like each other, approve of each other, and are willing to work together is vital to developing a strong team. Only such a team will ensure a smooth and effectively run office. As alluded to earlier, the applicant quite often will present a totally different personality at the front desk or in the waiting room than when with the interviewer. Therefore, after the second interview it is recommended that the employer again question any other staff person who has interacted with the applicant to give their honest opinion. Such input from other staff members will often bring traits and mannerisms to your attention that may have been missed in the interview. Another benefit of encouraging staff input is that when a staff member feels a degree of responsibility for the person being hired, that staff member is often more apt to make sure that person is made to feel welcome and will help ensure their success in their new position.

Hiring and Integrating the New Employee

Once the final decision is made, the process of hiring the new employee and establishing a successful relationship begins. As soon as the job offer is extended and accepted, a formal letter confirming the offer and the specifics of employment should be sent. Such a letter should describe the position offered, the beginning salary and benefits, the starting date, hours to be worked, and any other information deemed appropriate. Here, too, the employer should be careful to never imply a long-term relationship. The letter should request that the prospective employee confirm receipt of the letter and that all the information is correct and agreed to by calling the office by a given date.

When the new employee arrives on the first day, it is important that he or she immediately be made to feel welcome as a member of a great team. You (or a designated employee) should give the new employee a tour of the office. The new employee must be shown where to enter and leave the office, where to put personal belongings, how to clock in and out, where to eat lunch, etc. The tour should also include a review of the office floor plan, and a detailed description of what each room and each piece of equipment is used for. The new employee should then be introduced to and welcomed by every member of the staff present in the office.

Next, the new employee should be given a three-ringed binder containing the employee handbook, the job description, the operations manual for their position, and a section for staff meeting notes. Either yourself, or a delegated staff member, should review all aspects of the notebook with the employee, explaining each section of the handbook. Then, he or she should then be left alone to review the employee handbook. Once the employee has read the handbook, you should review each section and make sure the employee understands and agrees to the policies described. A written agreement to accept and abide by the policies described in the handbook should then be presented and signed by both the employee and the employer. A copy of the agreement is given to the employee and the original is placed in the employee's personnel file.

After review and acceptance of the employee handbook, the new employee's actual job description should be presented to them. Again the employee should be given sufficient time to review the description of the new job. Then, you (or a trusted staff member) should review the actual document with the new employee. After a review of the job description, the new employee should spend the rest of the day observing the actual functions of the position he or she will be performing.

On days two through four, either you or a trusted staff member should continue to review and reinforce the appropriate portions of the job description as they are being performed. During this time, the operations manual should be given to the new employee. Each day, the new employee should be given a new task to perform. They should perform it exactly as described by the operations manual, and be supervised closely by the office manager or yourself during this time. Slowly, the employee should be given more tasks to perform. By days 5 through 10, the new employee should have a working knowledge of each job function, and should be undertaking all aspects of the job description while still closely supervised. Within two weeks, the employee should be trained and capable of performing all procedures with a minimum of supervision and coaching.

During the first month, it is critical that you or someone in a supervisory capacity pays close attention to the new employee and tactfully corrects all mistakes and bad habits before they become established. At the same time, never forget the power and necessity of praising the new employee when he or she correctly performs their job. While correction and praise of an employee is appropriate at any time during employment, it is particularly important during the first month or two.

A new employee is a major investment in your office. This employee will play an important role in making the practice effective and efficient. A properly selected and trained employee plays a key role in helping the practice to reach its full potential. An unqualified or untrained employee, on the other hand, can be an anchor holding the practice back, preventing growth and limiting service to the community and the world. Finding the right people is a critical step in developing the type of practice you desire. Select employees carefully. Train and support them in every aspect of their jobs. A good employee may be the single most important investment doctors make in their practices.

Step 2-3: Coaching Your Dream Team

Once the staff is hired and in place, your leadership skills will mold these individuals into a team dedicated to the vision and mission of your practice. Leadership is a progressive, ongoing effort that will enlist support and motivate the individuals you have surrounded yourself with. These individuals will help you realize your ideal and the successful attainment of your practice mission.

To do this, you must have a vision of what the practice will be, and then communicate that vision to the staff. If done successfully, each member of the staff will know their role in the office, how their role furthers the common vision, and as such, will be self-motivated to do their job with minimal oversight. Essential to this is the consistent communication necessary to form such a team.

Weekly staff meetings will provide the forum for ongoing communications. It has been said that when two minds come together for a common purpose, a third mind is formed from such a relationship. No longer are there just two individual minds seeking a common end, but now three. This is called "synergy." Nowhere can this law be utilized more effectively than with your staff. Staff meetings are a time to ask questions, discuss problems, and to consider improvements in policies and procedures. It is also a wonderful opportunity to reinforce the mission of the practice, to set goals, and to congratulate, encourage, and praise.

Great care must be taken to include every member of the staff in such a meeting. You must remember that the staff meeting is a meeting of the staff…not a "doctor" meeting. Although you must provide leadership in the office, you must also listen to and gather information from each member of the staff. Staff meetings are a time to get ideas from your staff, to find out what is happening outside of the adjusting room—

Staff Meeting Agenda

Date: _____ Week Ending: _____

Highlights Of Last Meeting
1. _____
2. _____
3. _____

Review Of New Patients

	Patient	MAP Y	MAP N	Finances Cash	Finances Ins.	Remarks
1.	_____	☐	☐	☐	☐	_____
2.	_____	☐	☐	☐	☐	_____
3.	_____	☐	☐	☐	☐	_____
4.	_____	☐	☐	☐	☐	_____
5.	_____	☐	☐	☐	☐	_____
6.	_____	☐	☐	☐	☐	_____

Re-Activated Established Patients

	Patient	MAP Y	MAP N	Finances Cash	Finances Ins.	Remarks
1.	_____	☐	☐	☐	☐	_____
2.	_____	☐	☐	☐	☐	_____
3.	_____	☐	☐	☐	☐	_____

Review Of Past Week

Statistical Review:

New Patient Inquiries: _____   Scheduled New Patients: _____   New Patients: _____

Scheduled Visits: _____   Missed Appointments: _____   Missed Apts %: _____

Interrupted/ In completed MAPs:
1. _____ 3. _____
2. _____ 4. _____

Missed Payments: (This Week):
1. _____ 3. _____
2. _____ 4. _____

Goals & Projections

	New Pts	Pt Visits	Re-activations	Services	Collection %
Last Wk:	___	___	___	___	___
Next Wk:	___	___	___	___	___

Strategy Review Of The Week

Topic: _____ Requested By: _____

Summary: _____
_____
_____

Sample Form: **Staff Meeting Agenda**

on the front lines of the practice. At the same time, you must be careful not to make spontaneous procedural changes during the staff meeting. Before making important decisions about things that will impact the staff, patients, and practice, you should always take stock of the situation and carefully think it through.

Staff meetings simply have to be positive. This is not the place to criticize or reprimand. It is a time, however, to hold people accountable and provide support and encouragement when job functions are not being successfully performed. Discussion of reinforcement and rededication to the goals of the practice is always an important element of the weekly staff meeting, for which you need to preplan your agenda.

To further enhance the daily communications between you and your staff it is critical that you pay close attention to any new employees and correct all mistakes and bad habits before they become established. The front desk daily report provides just such a mechanism. This form should be completed and given to the doctor at the end of each day. It provides the doctor daily feedback on the day's activities and gives vital information on patients and follow-up telephone calls that should be made at the end of the day.

Most importantly, it provides a brief window of opportunity for you to thank and acknowledge your CA and the valuable assistance that he or she has provided. At the same time, it is an opportunity for the CA to advise you of any detail requiring special attention as a result of the day's activities.

Step 2-4: Things Aren't Always as They Seem—the "Phantom" CA

Early in practice, it may seem difficult to justify the cost of employing staff to answer phones and to process patients. It is especially hard when the practice has only a few patients and little actual work to be done. Still, it is vitally important for the doctor and the practice to put forward an appearance of being professional, successful, and yes...staffed.

Today's public has come to expect several important qualities and characteristics in a successful professional practice. Patients do not expect to see a successful doctor alone in the office—making appointments, collecting fees, typing insurance forms, and mopping the floor. Practicing without a CA may challenge many of these predetermined expectations to the point that the patient may actually develop doubts and uncertainty about your skills and abilities. Such uncertainty will usually generate a lack of confidence in both you and the practice, and will insidiously affect every aspect of patient management and practice growth.

Besides the obvious doubts, many patients, regardless of gender, may simply not be comfortable being alone in the office with just the doctor when no one else is present. It makes no difference whether you are male or female; the lack of another person in the office leaves you vulnerable for allegations of business and/or sexual improprieties. For this reason alone, you must always have a staff person present whenever patients are in the office.

For new practices, however, it may not be cost-efficient or even affordable to hire a full-time staff person until the patient load and the income can support such an investment. In situations where you cannot afford or justify a staff person, you may set up the office to give patients the impression that a full-time staff person is actually on hand. Such an illusion will convey the appearance that your practice is mature, profitable, and generally what the public expects. The "phantom" CA is a simple, inexpensive, effective way to address all of these considerations. If set up correctly, it gives the impression that there is a CA in the office, answering the telephone, and that you are not practicing alone.

The phantom CA concept works because of a combination of the "call forwarding" and "smart-ring" or "signal-calling" options available through the telephone companies. These features are usually minimally priced and so as not to raise the overall costs of the telephone bill all that much. The most important element of this system involves the efforts of a dedicated friend or family member and the effective utilization of block-booking techniques.

To set up the phantom CA system, you first have to identify someone who can to stay at home (or at any other remote location) during the late morning and early afternoon to professionally answer the telephone and book patients. The ideal person should have a personal interest in the practice's success and will perform these services for a minimal amount of pay (or for free)—maybe your spouse, or a relative who has an interest in your success. Or, this may be an ideal job for someone who is physically handicapped or who is simply near a phone for most of the day but cannot work full-time outside the home. Even if you must pay for this service, the amount will be minimal compared to that of a full-time employee. But remember, never sacrifice professionalism and a good telephone voice in the person who will be answering your phone and representing your practice.

Once this person has been found, the office telephone should be equipped with "call forwarding" and both (the office and remote) telephones should be set up with "smart-ring." By setting the remote phone to have a distinctive ring, the person at the remote location will know when incoming calls are being forwarded from the office and can answer them appropriately. The phantom CA should be trained in proper telephone techniques and etiquette and should answer as if actually sitting at the reception desk in the office. The caller will not know the difference.

Next, you will hire a part-time staff person (or possibly two) who will be scheduled to actually work in the office two to four hours a day to begin, i.e., the first two hours in the morning and the last two in the evening. These are the most preferred times for patients to come to the office and a front desk CA is needed for these times. The hours may be increased or another person hired as the patient load of the practice increases.

As above, the best person for this part-time, in-office position would be a spouse, relative or someone else who has an interest in the success of the practice. A work-release high school student who will come to the office and work for less than a full-time employee is also a viable option. You may find a work-release student by contacting the counselor of your local high school. Such students usually work for minimum wage and, besides being paid, are graded and receive school credit for their work in your office, therefore more likely to be conscientious and do a good job.

To make the phantom CA system work properly, you and your phantom CA will utilize a dual appointment book system and must communicate with each other as entries are made. Most important to making this procedure a success is to utilize block-booking procedures. By booking patients into blocks in the early morning and late afternoon, you may then hire a part-time CA, (or two) for just those hours. Their first responsibility will be to call the phantom CA and transfer the names of patients who have been booked into the office appointment book. Thus, you and your staff will know who will be coming in that afternoon and the following days. Not only does this system give you the ability to have a CA present when there are patients in the office, but it also gives patients the impression that the practice is strong and growing because of the full waiting room during these times.

Block booking for morning and afternoon hours also gives you the opportunity to leave the office from time to time to meet people, speak at noon luncheons, or to perform other practice building procedures in your community. But remember, you should discipline yourself to only leave the office for a specific practice-related reason. If you do leave the office during the day, carry a cell phone or a beeper so you may be summoned back to the office in case of an emergency. The afternoon CA should be scheduled to begin work at least 30 minutes prior to the first scheduled patient, and if you are out of the office, you should return at this time also. This gives the CA ample time to call the phantom CA and "download" the updated schedule of the late morning and early afternoon callers.

When the appointment book becomes full enough to begin booking patients during the late morning or over the lunch hour, a full-time CA can be added and afforded. The phantom CA concept is a wonderful way for a new practice to appear successful and allows you to protect yourself while saving valuable startup dollars. The new practice should utilize this procedure for as long is possible, filling the blocked times to capacity before extending the hours of the morning and/or afternoon CA.

By using the phantom CA concept, even the newest practice can employ a CA from the very first day the practice is open. While the new practice may not have the resources to employ a full-time assistant, almost any practice can give the impression of having a full-time person. A doctor should work alone only as a last resort. Right or wrong, a professional who has (or appears to have) a staff adheres more closely to the standards that the community expects from a successful, competent professional. Conforming to such expectations will significantly and positively impact the growth and success of the practice.

Conclusion

Developing and maintaining an efficient, effective, and dedicated staff is the first step in building your ideal practice. Therefore, it is also the most important managerial skill that every successful doctor must develop. This skill especially consists of having the intuitive ability to select and to surround yourself with effective people. Placing effective "help wanted" advertisements, efficient and effective interviewing, and making a fact-based, yet intuitive decision will fill your practice with good people. Initial time spent developing job descriptions, operations manuals, and employee handbooks are as important as any management duty undertaken, and will be time invested that will save many more hours in the years to come. Continued refining of these documents will ensure that the practice continues to stay on the cutting edge of staff development and management. Most importantly, continued attention to the effectiveness of these documents will set the stage for many years of stress-free staff and practice management.

Leading and motivating your staff on a daily basis is more difficult than creating employment documents, yet infinitely more important. This is an ongoing function of anyone managing a practice. Clear and concise communication of your primary objective is key to leading your staff toward building the practice. Communicating your purpose and your vision will help you to become a strong leader and result in the people you have surrounded yourself with aligning themselves with you.

You will never build your practice alone. It is your staff and those you surround yourself with who will, to a great extent, determine your success in making your dream come true. Being a leader in your own practice is much like being a magnet. You will attract similarly charged individuals with an invisible, yet irresistible power. Then, you will consistently and effortlessly pull them in the desired direction. But, if you have selected people who are not properly aligned, not similarly charged, as you and your vision, they will just as surely be repelled. Both are fundamental laws of magnetism, and will result in the expected result every time. Remember that it is okay to repel those who are not aligned with you. In fact, it is necessary. Recognize it and use it to your advantage. The hiring and training process that we have described above will help you to do just that.

In the end, always keep in mind that you are the leader in the office. It is an everyday, all-day job; you may never abdicate or delegate these responsibilities.

Key Points

- Job descriptions provide order and delineate positional functions and responsibilities for the performance of all vital activities in a systematic and orderly fashion.
- The operations manual is a document that essentially takes every single function described in the job description and says "this is how we do it here." It is the office's official "how-to-do-it" guide.
- The employee handbook is the employer's tool for establishing the rules, employment policies, and guidelines for dress and employee behavior.
- It cannot be emphasized enough that hiring people who like each other, approve of each other, and who are willing to work together is vital to developing a strong team.
- A properly selected and trained employee plays a key role in helping the practice reach its full potential. An unqualified or untrained employee, on the other hand, can be an anchor holding the practice back.
- Staff meetings are a time to ask questions, discuss problems, and to consider improvements in policies and procedures. It is also a wonderful opportunity to reinforce the mission of the practice, to set goals, and to congratulate, encourage, and praise.
- Patients do not expect to see a successful doctor alone in the office—making appointments, collecting fees, typing insurance forms, and mopping the floor.
- You will never build your practice alone. It is your staff and those who surround you that will, to a great deal, determine your success in making your dream come true.

Solution 3

Devise Systems for Success and Stability

Developing and refining key procedures into specific systems that will enable your practice to run smoothly and efficiently is a process borne of identifying the specific objectives and developing quantified tactics to meet these objectives. Such tactics fall into two critical categories. The first are those special tactics required for the practice to function in a controlled manner and the second are the, policies, procedures, and tactics that will encourage long-term practice growth.

The initial step in developing the special control systems that will put your practice on autopilot is to identify each objective that needs to be achieved for the practice to fulfill its own special mission. The best way to do this is to have each staff person keep a journal for a few days of everything they do on a daily basis. Each function undertaken by the doctor and staff will reveal their own ultimate objective or desired end result. It is then the doctor's job to interpret these activities and determine their true objectives. Recognition and interpretation of each activity is also a good ongoing subject for staff meetings, bringing each employee into the process of practice development.

After identifying each practice objective, the next step is to shape systematic means of achieving those objectives. This will probably be the most time-consuming aspect of the entire process, because here is where you develop the special tactics as to how you want your staff to meet their objectives,—written in as great a detail as possible. These tactics, policies, and procedures will eventually fill your practice procedures manual.

The final step is quantifying the achieved results. Without keeping statistics on a daily, weekly, monthly, and annual basis, you will have no idea as to the effectiveness of your policies, procedures, and tactics in meeting your practice objectives.

The following systems are just a few examples of how you can handle a few of the most critical objectives in your office:

First, you will quickly identify two of the most time-consuming activities in as the movement of the patient from the reception area to the adjusting rooms, and pulling and filing patient folders for each visit. Both are time intensive for your staff, and therefore lead to inefficiency and higher overhead.

Having identified these two objectives, you can then begin to develop a system for satisfying both. For instance, using a patient information (PI) card system and numbered room system may satisfy both objectives. The clipboard system will efficiently move your patients through the office. At the same time, this system places all of the information needed to process both the new and the routine visit at everyone's fingertips. Your staff won't need to pull and rummage through piles of paperwork in a patient's file that is not needed for each individual visit.

The patient scheduling and the case management plan is another system that will allow you to meet your patient management objectives. By identifying the need to keep the patient scheduled with future visits that will comply with the doctor's recommended frequency of care, you will easily see that creating multiple appointments for the patient at one time, will enable the staff to effectively manage your patient's schedule of care. Effectively designed and executed, a system of making multiple appointments at a time, should produce the desired results of enhancing patient compliance and appointment without being extremely staff intensive.

These are just two examples of tactics that can be developed to successfully and efficiently reach the objectives identified above. Such systems must be employed for virtually every function of a successful practice. This may be an ongoing procedure, but it will be rewarding as you see your systems effectively put into place and your staff and practice become efficient, profitable, and professional.

The most important parallel procedure in developing and maintaining a successful practice is the systematic tracking of all the various statistics that will allow the effective manager to monitor and predict the effectiveness of staff and all other systems. Then, once you have identified all of your daily practice objectives and designed systems and special tactics, you need to know if your systems, policies, and procedures are effective in reaching your objectives with the desired result.

Quantifying the effectiveness of each procedure requires knowledge of both past and present indicators and the trends they reveal. This is so important to building the practice of your dreams that an entire section has been devoted to the subject later on. The following sections will have a major impact on those statistical evaluations of your practice.

Step 3-1: Sharpen Your Message and Focus Your Communication

Day in and day out, we are called upon to deliver the same information to many different patients. If you ever have played the childhood game of "telephone'" you know that each time something is repeated it changes slightly…almost imperceptibly. The same is true with you and your staff. Each time you tell someone about your practice, the message changes. You may have initially planned and scripted all of the information you want your patients to have, but sooner or later, the messenger tires of the message.

The creation and use of specific personalized office brochures can effectively transmit the vital information that all patients should be given. These will sharpen your message and should support you and your staff's verbal conveyance of all important information to patients. Personalized office brochures also serve as impressive and effective tools for practice marketing.

The first brochure should be simply a "practice" brochure. A practice brochure should be an "about our office" brochure. It should give the current patient, prospective patient, and referring patient all of the information necessary to be familiar with you, your practice, and your basic policies. Typically, such a brochure should contain such specifics as: personal and professional information about you, your philosophy of practice, a brief introduction to chiropractic, location and directions to the office, how to call for and make appointments, office hours, plus anything else you may deem appropriate. This brochure is an important element in the internal marketing efforts of the practice. It should be warmly written and inviting.

A Welcome to Our Office brochure is a great way to greet new patients, welcome them to the office, and give them more information about specific policies and procedures of the practice. This brochure should include additional information about the philosophy of the practice, specific information about certain office policies, and a picture of you and possibly even your staff. A brief introduction of each staff member and how they will assist the patient will familiarize the patient with the staff. This brochure may be given to each new patient to read prior to initial consultation, or mailed to the new patient along with a "Welcome to Our Office" letter.

Next, may be a Financial Policy brochure. When your policies and procedures are displayed in ink, it is much easier for patients to understand your policies and your staff to enforce them.

Most important, every chiropractic office should have a Subluxation/Adjustment brochure that clearly and succinctly describes the Vertebral Subluxation Complex, as well as its many causes and its adverse effects on health and adaptation. It is most effectively used as a warm-up to the case report. By giving this brochure to the patient at the end of the first visit to read before returning for the second visit case review, you set the stage and improve the patient's concepts of chiropractic. Its primary objective is to indoctrinate the patient with the basic concepts of chiropractic, dis-ease, health, and wellness.

Although you may find reasons for additional brochures, the effective development of these three brochures is critical. They will be useful in adequately representing your practice, and to educate your patients. They will have a huge impact on your ability to present a consistently good image of your practice, and to educate your patients about your office policies and chiropractic.

Step 3-2: PI Cards—Eliminate the Paper Chase While Staying on Track

Daily pulling of entire file folders is tedious, inefficient, and because of the size of some patient files, it could also be dangerous to your staff. I am still amazed that, in this day and age, offices are still using systems that require the staff to waste time by pulling and filing entire patient folders on each visit. In reality, to properly service the patient on a routine visit, the doctor may need only one—possibly two—pieces of information contained in the file. If you are pulling daily files in your office, I challenge you to do a time study on how much time your CA spends just getting out and putting away file folders. If you are not yet in practice, take my word for it. It is a waste of time and counterproductive. With proper planning and design of your system, this activity is simply not necessary.

Streamlining this procedure requires one basic form, the patient information (PI) card. This single form is simple to integrate into both new and existing chiropractic offices. Over the years it will save the staff hundreds of hours of work, and the doctor thousands of dollars. The patient information (PI) card is an 8½- by-11-inch (bi-folded) document printed on card stock. Although it does not replace the patient's file folder, it does replace having the CA pull and file the entire folder on every patient visit. More importantly, it contains all of the information necessary for you to manage and adjust the patient, using one document, thus avoiding the massive paper shuffle that usually accompanies the typical office visit when the entire patient folders are pulled and filed.

The real advantage of the PI card is that it contains all of the pertinent patient information in one place. Properly designed, the PI card contains specific places for entering every aspect of the patient's personal and clinical information. Personal information such as the patient's name, address, marital status, etc. should be placed at the top of the card for ease of recognition and filing. A special area for the graphic identification of the patient's entrance complaints consists of an ante-

♦ 7 Solutions for Building Your Proactive Chiropractic Practice ♦

PATIENT INFORMATION

- Patient Name:
- Case #:
- Age: M/S/W/D
- Date of Birth:
- Phone:
- Phone:
- Referred By:
- Coverage:
- Spouse:
- Address:
- Business:
- Occupation:
- Insurance Co.
- Other:

CONSULTATION SYNOPSIS

- Complaint:
- Duration:
- Traumas:
- Prev. Drs:
- Opinions:
- Prv. Care:
- Env. Links:
- Lifestyle:
- Hereditary:
- Other:

DIAGNOSIS
ICDA Codes | Date

REFERRED PATIENTS
Name | Date

INITIAL SUBLUXATION EXAMINATION

POSTURE & MOVEMENT

Postural Analysis
- Head Tilt ☐ Lt ☐ Rt +____
- Shoulder Tilt ☐ Lt ☐ Rt +____
- Pelvic Tilt ☐ Lt ☐ Rt +____

Weight Bearing
- Weight: ____
- Distr: ☐ Lt ☐ Rt +____
- Stability: ____

Lumbar Ranges of Motion

	Degrees	Pain
Flexion	/90	
Extension	/45	
L. Rot.	/30	
R. Rot.	/30	
L. Flex.	/30	
R. Flex.	/30	

Cervical Range of Motion

	Degrees	Pain
Flexion	/45	
Extension	/45	
L. Rot.	/80	
R. Rot.	/80	
L. Flex.	/45	
R. Flex.	/45	

NERVE SYSTEM

Reflexes

	Lt.	Rt.
Biceps		
Triceps		
Extensors		
Patellar		
Achilles		

Neuro-Ortho Testing
- For Comp:
- Max Comp:
- Sh Dep:
- Distract:
- Valsalva:
- Cranial Nerves:
- Dermatomes:
- Toe Walk:
- Heel Walk:
- Rhomberg:

Observation / Notes / Other:
____
____
____

MUSCLE & STRENGTH

Circumference

	Lt.	Rt.
Thigh		
Calve		
Biceps		
Forearm		

Neuro-Ortho Testing
- SotoHall:
- S.L.R:
- Braggard:
- Leg Drop:

Dynamometer
- Lt Hand ____
- Rt Hand ____

Vitals
- Blood Pressure:
  - Lt ____/____
  - Rt ____/____
- VBA:
- Subclavian:
- Carotid:
- Heart:

PALAPATORY EXAMINATION

MS	TP	SP	TP	MS
		OC		
		C1		
		C2		
		C3		
		C4		
		C5		
		C6		
		C7		
		T1		
		T2		
		T3		
		T4		
		T5		
		T6		
		T7		
		T8		
		T9		
		T10		
		T11		
		T12		
		L1		
		L2		
		L3		
		L4		
		L5		

Sacrum

Sample Form: **Patient Information (PI) Card, front**

◆ Devise Systems for Success and Stability ◆

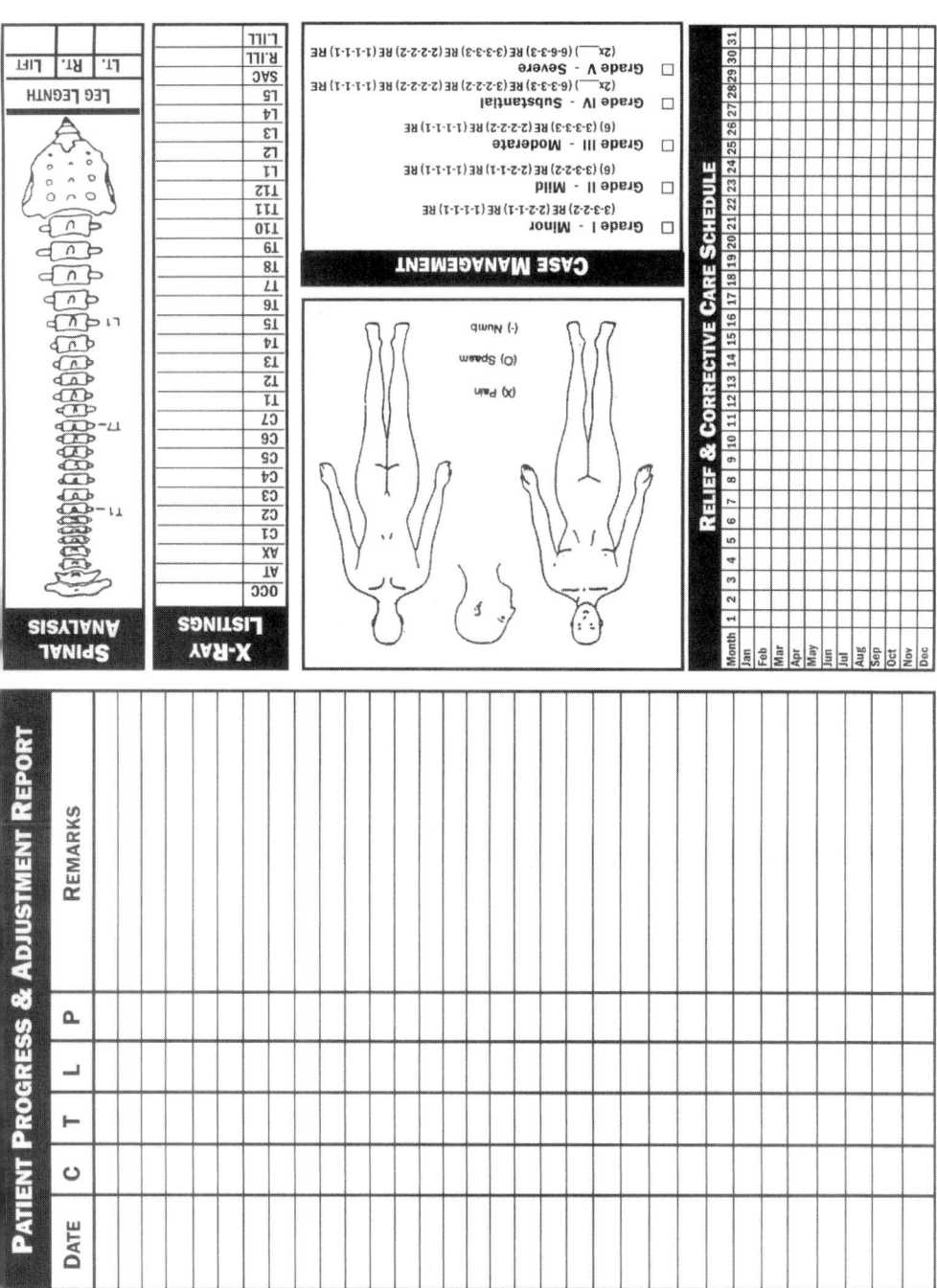

Sample Form: **Patient Information (PI) Card, back**

rior and posterior full body graphic similar to that appearing on the patient's case information sheet.

On the card should be a typed synopsis of the patient's initial consultation and case history. The information will come from the new patient consultation worksheet that you will complete during the new patient consultation. The CA should transfer this information onto the PI card after the patient's initial visit. An area for you to denote the important examination and x-ray findings or other clinical analytical findings is important and helpful in the day-to-day management of the patient. Also included should be an area in which you may list the initial diagnosis and subsequent revisions as the patient improves.

Special technique notes may be given priority space on the card. Such an entry may be used to alert you to any contraindications to specific techniques or as to what your technique and adjusting plan may be. Most importantly, and given the most space, should be a panel for you to record the patient's objective and subjective findings on each visit. Here you will also record the adjusting history of the patient, with visit-by-visit analysis if indicated by your particular technique.

By including the patient's subluxation listings and various spinal analysis findings, you now have a complete view of the patient's case and understand the full complexities on only one document.

The folded size (5 by 8½ inches) of the patient information card is important because it allows the card to fit into the file boxes typically sold for storage of the ledger cards for pegboard systems. This compact tray permits ease of filing, physical security for the cards, and accessibility for the CA. The best reason for incorporating the PI card is that pulling the entire patient file on each visit can now be avoided. Now, all of the patient's financial records, x-rays, and other documents that are not essential to the patient's visit-to-visit paperwork may be left secure in the file cabinets.

To help standardize the recommendation process and the multiple appointing of the active patient, a listing of the three or four most commonly recommended case plans may also be indicated on the card. Once this is accomplished, your prescribed schedule of care is now ready for you to check off once your clinical deliberations have brought you to a conclusion as to the recommendations indicated by each particular case. You will quickly find that this box, with its check-off recommenda-

♦ Devise Systems for Success and Stability ♦

tions, will speed up your decision-making process and improve the communication of the case plan to the CA who will be scheduling the necessary appointments.

Another feature of the PI card that will significantly improve patient scheduling and help you to develop more effective management of the patient's recommended care is to include a 12-month calendar. Such a calendar will show all future appointments and will provide effective control and tracking of the patient's visits. By using a calendar on your PI card, you will be able to see at a glance where the patient is on the recommended case plan and when reevaluations may be coming up. Such a clear overview of the entire case plan will tremendously help both doctor and staff in the day-to-day management of the case.

Best of all, with all of the above information contained on one piece of paper, the PI cards are easily copied when information needs to be sent to insurance companies, attorneys, and various other outside parties.

The well-designed PI card is the single most effective tool in managing your patients that can be incorporated into a chiropractic office. Design this card well and it will become a great investment in the practice's growth and success.

Step 3-3: Keep Everyone on the Same Page—Use a Service Slip

For the staff to schedule and reappoint efficiently, for the patient's clinical case to be managed effectively, and for proper charging of fees on each visit, a foolproof system of communication between the front desk and the doctor is critical. At every point of patient interaction, every visit, the doctor and the CA have a fail-safe means of constantly communicating with each other. The most efficient means of communicating what services were rendered, what charges were incurred at each visit, and the doctor's order for when the patient should return is by using a service slip at each visit. The service slip concept is both simple in design and effective in use. By using a form that gives the doctor the ability to record what services were rendered to the patient on each visit, as well as any special orders for continued management of the case, the CA can always handle the patient processing correctly.

Also, by including all of the information needed for the patient to submit their charges directly to the insurance company for reimbursement, the service slip can also serve as an insurance "super bill" thus alleviating the need for the CA to process insurance forms for the patient.

In order for patients to receive reimbursement without your staff having to assist them, be sure to include your license number, federal identification number, and any other appropriate numbers that will facilitate reimbursement for the patient on the form. The body of this form should be a listing of all of the services rendered in the office, as well as the appropriate CPT codes. The form should also contain an area for you or a staff person to record the patient's current or updated diagnosis code for that visit.

Also, to better communicate your orders for follow-up care between the adjusting rooms and the front desk, there should be a specific space on the slip for you to note when the patient should return for future care. The return visit should always be noted even if the patient is currently scheduled on a multiple appointment program. The reason for this is simple yet powerful: If you

Sample Form: **Service Slip**

Service Slip & Insurance Statement

MEYER CHIROPRACTIC OFFICES
8100 W US Hwy 20 - Box 1025
SHIPSHEWANA, IN 46565
(260) 768-7806

Date of Service: ___/___/___
Patient:_____
Diagnosis:_____

OFFICE VISITS
☐ 99202 New Patient Exam
☐ 99212 Established Patient Exam
☐ 99242 Office Visit, Consultation

PROCEDURES
☐ 98941 Spinal Adjustment
    (___) Adults
    (___) Youth
    (___) Child
    (___) Family
☐ 98943 Extra-spinal Adjustment
☐ _____ Other:_____

DISPENSARY SUPPLIES
☐ _____ _____

RADIOLOGY
☐ 72010 Spine Entire (___ views)
☐ 72040 Spine Cervical (2 views)
☐ 72050 Spine Cervical (4 views)
☐ 72070 Spine Thoracic (2 views)
☐ 72100 Spine, Lumbar (2 views)
☐ _____ Other:_____

PT TO RETURN:	TOTAL
	PREVIOUS BALANCE
	PAYMENT
———	NEW BALANCE

NEXT APPOINTMENT:_____

MICHAEL S. MEYER, D.C.
FEDERAL ID #XX-XXXXXXX
Form - 03   INDIANA LICENSE NO.: XXXXXXXX

can discipline yourself to check the patient's progress thorough his or her recommended schedule of appointments, and then record the next visit on the service slip, both you and your CA are thereby reminded to verbally reinforce the next scheduled visit to the patient.

Such reinforcement shows the patient that both doctor and the staff are serious about the patient's recommended care and that the doctor is aware of the patient's progress through their multiple appointment series. Knowing that the doctor is constantly monitoring their schedule will have a positive impact on patients' maintaining their care, and on the percentage of patients who miss their appointments in general.

The procedure is simple. The service slip is placed on the patient's clipboard along with the patient information card and sent to the adjusting room with the patient. After completing the day's visit, you will check off the services performed with the proper CPT code listed and record for the CA when the next appointment should be made.

If the patient is filing their own insurance, the CA should record the patient's current ICDA diagnostic code numbers onto the slip, charges for the day, and finish processing the patient. The CA can then explain to the patient that if they wish to file for any insurance benefits, they should simply complete the patient's section of their insurance form and attach the service slips to the physician's section. Properly designed, the service slip should contain all of the information necessary for the patient to file for and receive reimbursement.

Just a note of caution: If the practice has accepted an assignment of benefits for this patient and is waiting for payment by the insurance company, the CA should *never* record the ICDA code numbers on this slip. With such information, the unscrupulous patient can easily submit these forms for reimbursement and receive payments that rightfully should have been sent directly to your office.

Step 3-4: Systematize Your Case Management Plan and Appointment Scheduling

Case management plans (CMP) and multiple appointment programs (MAP) are powerful ways to build and add tremendous stability to the practice. They are also fantastic tools in helping patients manage their journey back to health and wellness. It is a procedure that encourages booking several appointments at one time for new patients during the initial three phases of care. Based on the doctor's recommendations for the patient's care (that will be further described in a later section) the MAP series is the actual manifestation of the recommendations that you have made to the patient during the case review. Properly explained and designed, these appointments will be anticipated by the patient. In addition, the patient will appreciate the advance reserving of convenient times.

Patient Benefits

There are many benefits to the patient as well as to the office when all new patients are placed on a series of appointments. These benefits include:

1. It allows patients to schedule their lives around the appointments previously committed to in your office. People naturally schedule their lives around previous standing appointments. Therefore, if a patient has an appointment scheduled in your office in advance, all subsequent appointments made elsewhere (other doctors, haircuts, social engagements, etc.) are typically made around their preexisting appointments.

2. It increases continuity of care and reduces patient attrition. If a patient who is on a preset series of appointments, misses an appointment and cannot be recalled, they will automatically have another subsequent appointment scheduled. It increases efficiency and decreases stress and redundant activities at the front desk.

3. The patient, who already has future appointments made in advance, does not have to stop at the front desk and make a new appointment at the end of each visit. This will significantly increase the efficiency of the front desk by relieving the CA of scheduling an appointment on every visit. As a patient leaves, a smile, a wave, and a goodbye from the CA is much easier than booking a new appointment after each visit.

4. It reserves times convenient to the patient, reducing the visit-by-visit lottery of available times that might fit into the patient's schedule.

◆ Devise Systems for Success and Stability ◆

5. It improves your ability to manage the case. You will always know at a glance exactly where the patient is in their schedule of recommended care. Such knowledge will greatly increase your ability to properly manage the patient's case from visit to visit.

6. It helps the staff to automatically schedule atypical visits and procedures. In fact, it is important that any unusual visits with additional procedures are automatically scheduled at appropriate times and well in advance. Pre-scheduling such procedures will prevent oversight of necessary reevaluations, consultations, x-ray updates, or exercise programs.

7. It is extremely effective in enhancing practice stability. Case management plans are essential for the stability of the practice. If this procedure is being properly performed, the appointment book should be relatively full four to six weeks in advance.

    This practice stability is born from the fact that patients only have to make one decision as to whether or not they will continue with care. Most significant in this process is that the decision is made at the time when the patient has all the information necessary to make an informed decision and when that information is fresh in their minds—at, or immediately following, the case review. Once a series of appointments is set and accepted, the patient will not have to continually decide whether they will reappoint for another visit or not.

8. The multiple appointment system allows for effective tracking of patient compliance and necessary follow-up. Used as an important discussion topic during staff meetings, any patient who discontinues or gets off their recommended series of appointments will not fall through the cracks. Reporting and discussing such patients will allow the staff and doctor to decide how to most effectively institute an appropriate course of action to preserve the continuity of the patient's care.

Step 3-5: Create Specific Procedures for Reappointing Your Current Patients

The most effective system to keep the patient on the recommended course of care is accomplished face-to-face with the patient at the end of the appointment. For this reason, both you and your front desk staff must have systematic procedures and work together closely to impress upon the patient the importance of correction, wellness, and the long-term healthful aspects of chiropractic care. The effectiveness of you and your CA in scheduling future follow-up visits will greatly aid in reducing the amount of recall and reactivation needed. Although much of the motivation for patient follow-through does rest with the doctor, most of the actual execution lies with the CA.

The real success of patient management is the degree to which the doctor has initially provided understandable and logical recommendations. Still, in most cases, at the end of each and every visit, the doctor should tell, or reinforce to, the patient when to return, and restate the reason why. Just as important as your degree of belief and certainty in your clinical abilities, you must have the same level of conviction and dedication to successfully realizing the objectives of the clinical care that you have recommended. If you have any doubts or lack of certainty as to the stated objectives, the patient's needs, or your ability to deliver for the patient, you will likely shirk the essential duty of reinforcing your recommendations. If so, patient follow-through will most assuredly suffer.

Anyone who has been in practice for any length of time understands that most patients need (and want) to be told how to take care of themselves. Telling patients when to return for their next visit is paramount to proper patient management and a duty for any conscientious doctor. Without continuity in patient care, obtaining maximum clinical results and the continued well-being of patients will not be effected

As a side note, I recommend you never get into the habit of only making recommendations for follow-up visits on even numbered weeks such as in increments of two-, four-, or six-week intervals. For some reason, many doctors fall into this pattern, and lose the flexibility to recommend more frequent visits (three-, five-, or seven-week intervals instead of four, six, or eight) if needed. In addition, we have found that patients seem to remember odd numbered week intervals better, thus helping to effect a lower missed appointment rate.

To communicate the patient's need for follow-up care, you must note the length of time between appointments on the patient's receipt and reinforce the reasons why they should return.

> **Doctor:** "Mrs. Jones, you need to continue your corrective care program and we will continue to monitor your progress So let's get that second cervical checked again in three weeks. In the meanwhile, be sure to do the exercises we discussed last week and avoid stress. Do you have any questions?"

When you release the patient, the CA must make the next appointment before the patient leaves the office for effective follow-up. The doctor's reinforcement of when and why to return, and the front desk's proper booking techniques, are the best way to prevent patients from leaving the office without a future appointment and drifting back to a subluxated life.

Often when the practice is extremely busy and staff has other pressing needs, it may seem easier for the CA to simply tell the patient they are due back in three weeks and let them leave without taking time to schedule another appointment. Such a casual approach is not only devastating for the practice, but it is a great disservice to the patient as well. Every effort should be made by the doctor to recommend a return date and by the CA to schedule a subsequent appointment when indicated.

As the scripts show, the actual wording used by the CA is extremely important. A common mistake often made by the CA is to tell the patient that the *doctor* "wants" or "needs" to see the patient in three weeks. Always keep in mind, the patient has the need—*not* the doctor.

Script

> **CA:** "The doctor noted that you will need to have your spine checked again in three weeks, Mrs. Jones. Would you prefer Tuesday the 18th or Wednesday the 19th? Okay...morning or afternoon?
>
> "Would you prefer first thing in the morning or later?
>
> "Sure...11:00 or 11:15 A.M.?"

By using the above "forcing technique," the CA now has the ability to effectively reschedule the departing patient, allowing the patient to be "forced" into the block-booking pattern desired by the CA. It is also extremely efficient in quickly bringing the patient to a day and time that will fit their schedule without a prolonged listing of available times.

Step 3-6: Develop a Procedure for the Declined Appointment

In your continuing efforts to help your patients maintain a healthy, abundant life by remaining subluxation-free, you need to develop systems to keep the patient "on the books" and maintaining their adjustments. Therefore, the goal of the front desk should be that every patient who leaves the office has an appointment for a return visit, unless the doctor specifies otherwise.

Some patients, however, periodically (or routinely) decline to make further appointments. These patients often only return when they are symptomatic. Some simply have scheduling difficulties. Young mothers and busy business people often fall into this category.

Often patients will say, "Let me check my schedule and call you back." Although these people may be wonderful patients who have every intention of returning within the recommended time frame, the pressures and responsibilities of life often interfere. Experience has shown that if patients do not get their appointments on the books (theirs as well as yours) they often will not obtain the care needed. Unfortunately, these patients and circumstances usually become known only at the front desk and the doctor has no idea these patients are not rescheduling their appointments. It is up to the doctor to understand that these situations commonly present themselves, and then, to create policies, procedures, and scripts. These special tactics will help the CA to encourage the patient to act in his or her own best interest, and to making specific plans for a return visit. Such a situation can be handled by:

> **CA**: "The doctor suggests that you have your nervous system checked again in three weeks. Can I reserve 11:00 on Tuesday the 14th for you?"
>
> **Patient:** "I'm not sure of my schedule."

CA: "Let's reserve that time for you anyway...I will write it in pencil and you can call me back if this does not work."

If the patient still declines to make an appointment, the CA should place the patient's name, phone number, and day of the recommended appointment on a Post-it note and stick it on the appropriate day in the appointment book. The patient should then be called within a few days of the recommended return date to schedule the appointment.

Step 3-7: Manage the Inevitable Missed Appointment

Missed appointments are frustrating, harmful to the patient's recovery, costly to the practice—and inevitable. The most common (and most ambiguous) breakdown in patient follow-through always begins with the missed appointment. If the patient has missed an appointment and is not contacted and rescheduled in a timely manner, they will experience a loss or a delay in the correction of their subluxation and its attending complex. Inevitably, such a setback in the patient's progress will be blamed on the doctor's inability to achieve the desired results or the ineffectiveness of chiropractic itself. Therefore, proper leadership on the part of the doctor, is so important that there must be specific policies, procedures, and oversight designed to properly address this problem.

Of course, it is the CA's responsibility to immediately identify the missed appointment and initiate the recall system to prevent the patient from getting off their recommended schedule of care, or worse yet, the patient prematurely discontinuing their current phase of care. Because the front desk CA is always the first person to deal with the "missed appointment," the CA potentially can have an incredible impact on the patient's health and future well-being. The recall of a missed appointment is a tremendously beneficial procedure for helping the patient follow the doctor's recommendations and experience the full value of their chiropractic care, and should receive a high degree of attention by the doctor.

We all realize that any alteration in frequency of visits or disruption of care can be devastating to the patient's improvement and subluxation eradication. Therefore, preventative measures can be most effective

Missed Appointment Log

WEEK ENDING ___/___/___

	Name	Phone	Hm	Wk	Date Missed	Date Re-Schd	Contact Date	Pt. Ref.	Schd Error	PH By
1.										
2.										
3.										
4.										
5.										
6.										
7.										
8.										
9.										
10.										
11.										
12.										
13.										
14.										
15.										
16.										
17.										
18.										
19.										
20.										

Special Notes:

Sample Form: **Missed Appointment Log**

◆ Devise Systems for Success and Stability ◆

in helping patients achieve the clinical results hoped for. In most cases, preventative measures such as telephone reminders, post cards reminders, and e-mail reminders can prove extremely effective in saving patients time, money, and, most importantly, needless pain and suffering.

In our decades of practice, we have seen repeatedly that when a patient has missed their appointment, the first 15 to 30 minutes are critical in contacting the patient and keeping them on schedule. Any patient who has apparently missed an appointment should be called exactly 15 minutes after the scheduled appointment time. If the patient cannot be reached, follow-up calls (same script) are made later in the day, or the next day if the patient is not reached.

Contacting the missed appointment should never be an adversarial or a confrontational situation. In fact, the secret to successfully recalling a missed appointment is to take all blame away from the patient and prevent the person from becoming defensive. A useful script may be as follows:

CA: "Mrs. Jones, please? Hi, Mrs. Jones, this is Carol from Dr. Meyer's office calling. Mrs. Jones, I'm sorry to bother you, but I may have made a mistake in my appointment book. Could you tell me when your next appointment is?"

At that point, the patient usually remembers he or she has just missed an appointment and will begin to apologize profusely. However, before the patient goes too far, the CA should assure the patient that they are still a loved and appreciated member of the practice, and that while it is understood that things like this happen, the doctor is most concerned with their progress and merely wants what is best for the patient:

CA: "Mrs. Jones, I understand. These things occasionally happen. Nevertheless, the doctor is concerned because (he or she) knows how important it is that you stay on schedule and not lose any of the correction you have made so far. We can see you yet today, and we can keep you on your schedule of care. In fact, we have time yet this morning or would this afternoon be better?"

If the patient refuses to make a new appointment, the CA should report it to the doctor at the end of the day for follow-up at his or her discretion.

Whether the patient is successfully rescheduled or not, the situation should always be recorded in the "progress notes" section of the PI card—preferably in red. Recording the transgression and the reason alerts and informs the doctor of a possible compliance problem and helps the doctor to successfully manage the patient at the next visit. Although it is the CA who must take the basic procedural steps necessary to contact and to reschedule the patient, it is always the doctor who must be "the enforcer." When the doctor sees the PI card and first becomes aware of the missed appointments, it is important that the doctor have a serious "heart-to-heart" discussion with the patient. The patient should be told that the doctor is aware of the breach, that missing appointments will severely retard or prevent the patient from enjoying the anticipated results, and that there are other patients who could have been booked during that time.

The bottom line is that such actions are not acceptable in your practice and future missed appointments cannot be tolerated and will result in the patient's being released or referred. "Hard-nosed" confrontation in this area is appropriate and often necessary. Not only the patient's welfare is on the line, but your practice and reputation as well. You must maintain control.

> *Note:* The CA must always record missed and canceled appointments on the patient information card, the reason for the miss (if known), as well as the rescheduled date. I recommend this be recorded in red ink. If a patient habitually misses appointments, the doctor may not realize it. If all missed appointments are recorded in red, it is easy for the doctor to quickly recognize and deal with such a problem. Likewise, a habitual "misser" seldom obtains the anticipated results. Such a record will quickly give the doctor the rationale for the lack of success when questioned by the patient or a third party.

Step 3-8: Contacting the Unscheduled Patient

From time to time, there may be patients who are not able to reschedule follow-up visits. There are also patients who may routinely return at unpredictable intervals. These may be the types of patients the doctor has simply given up on trying to place on a routine schedule. Although some of these may be good patients, this situation is to be avoided as much as possible. Continuing educational efforts are indicated for these patients, as it may reflect a breakdown in understanding or follow-through. Still, we know there will always be some patients who do have difficulty booking advance appointments or prefer to make their appointment as time and need allow.

The best way to handle these patients is for the doctor to write the letters "RAN" (return as needed) or "WC" (will call) on the patient's service slip and in the patient's progress notes for that date. The doctor should then record "three, five, or seven weeks." This represents the time interval in which the staff should follow up with the patient by telephone. In such an instance, the patient's name and phone number should be entered into a special section in the appointment book on the proper day, or into a patient call book for future contact.

When the indicated day arrives for the patient to be called, the CA should call the patient and make inquires into any changes in symptomatology, environment, or lifestyle, and offer an appointment. Quite often, the patient will volunteer to make an appointment at that time—even stating he or she had been meaning to call for an appointment. But if the patient is doing well, just the service attitude of a phone call will be appreciated and will help to maintain a strong relationship between the patient and the practice. The CA should remember that this is not necessarily a call to book an appointment, just to maintain contact with the patient and the patient's family. If the patient is doing well and does not schedule another appointment, the CA should end the call by asking the patient's permission to check with them again in the future. At that point, the CA should record the conversation on the patient's PI card, and schedule another call in roughly twice the time originally recommended.

Step 3-9: Systematically Recalling the Inactive Patient

Realistically, even the most effective and conscientious staff will not be able to reappoint everyone who should be. As a result, some patients fall through the cracks and need to be called and checked on from time to time. The periodic follow-up of inactive patients is truly one of the most caring services that a practice can perform. An effective recall system lets the patient know that they are not forgotten and that their doctor is concerned about the health and well-being of his or her patients—even those who have not been seen for some time.

Therefore, one of the most important functions of the CA is to make sure that patients are actively and effectively recalled. Inactive patients should be telephoned on the third, sixth, ninth, and twelfth month after their last visit. Most computer programs can provide a printout of these people and can easily be used as a worksheet.

Calling inactive patients is important for several reasons. It shows that your practice cares about them and their families. Often the patients will state that they have been meaning to call for an appointment, but have not gotten around to it. Proper recalling, with the right scripts and attitude, helps to build goodwill toward your office and maintains a bond with past patients.

To make your recall efforts as effective as possible, several factors should be considered:

Your odds of success are greatly enhanced if you routinely send reminder cards to patients at three-month intervals and then follow-up with a personal phone call from a staff member. While such cards are a gentle nudge to get the patient thinking about returning, they often don't totally motivate the patient to make the effort to call and make an appointment at that time. The card does, however, get the patient thinking about the fact that they are due for a checkup and possible adjustment, and that their doctor and staff are thinking about them.

Then, when they actually do get a call from their doctor's office, they are more apt to respond positively and schedule an appointment. A personal hand-written and signed message by the doctor on these cards (Such as "Hi, Jenny…How's the new puppy?" or something similar. Just keep it short and personal.) will also improve the patient's positive response. Use all three of the above strategies and the success is multiplied.

The recall is *not* being made to find out how the patient is doing and the caller should never ask, "How are you?" The reason is simple, most patients do not know how they truly are (on a clinical level) and the stock answer is always, "I am fine." If they are "fine," why do they need to make another appointment to see the doctor? Obviously, the CA should be trained to avoid asking patients this question—both on the phone and in person. Remember, the patient has no idea.

◆ Devise Systems for Success and Stability ◆

When a staff member is performing the recall procedures and patient contact is made, the CA should immediately identify himself or herself and the reason for the call.

> *CA:* "Hi, Mrs. Jones, this is Carol from Dr. Meyer's office. The doctor asked me to call you today to schedule you for your (3-, 6-, 9-, 12-month) nerve scan and subluxation assessment." (Pause for the patient to reply either in the negative or the affirmative.)

Then, the CA should state the office's policy for recall procedures and subsequent payment:

> *CA:* "Mrs. Jones, the doctor is so committed to keeping our patients subluxation-free and their nerve systems functioning properly that when you come in, the doctor will do a computerized nerve and muscle scan, as well as check your posture, weight bearing, and ranges of spinal motion. If you have held your adjustment and no correction is necessary, there is no charge for this service.
>
> "If you are subluxated again, and you do need an adjustment, the doctor might be able to correct it at that time, or at least schedule for a return visit."

The CA should never ask the patient if they "would like" to make an appointment. Instead, assume that they will, and offer the patient a choice of two different days.

> *CA:* "Would you prefer next Tuesday or Wednesday?"

Then proceed to book the appointment as usual.
If the patient hesitates or declines the appointment, the CA should add:

> *CA:* "Mrs. Jones, just as with your teeth and eyes, periodic checkups are important. Because your spine will often 'drift back' to its old abnormal position, and before you realize it, it may be too late.
>
> "The biggest benefit of these checkups is that if you are developing any problems, we can catch them before you end up like you were when you first came in.

"And, again, if you are okay and don't need an adjustment, there will be no charge for the checkup.

"Are you sure we can't get you in next week?"

If the patient further declines reappointment, the CA should graciously thank the patient for their time, and extend a warm invitation for them to call the office anytime they may need to, and that the doctor and staff will look forward to that day, when it comes.

As most of us know, the dental professional has been extremely successful in setting up effective recall procedures that patients have come to expect and rely on. It has become a rewarding program for most offices and a wonderful service for the patient. Unfortunately, most patients take the position that "If my doctor is not going to worry about my health, then why should I?" To this attitude, we respond, "Okay, we *will* take that responsibility." We show our concern for our patients and our passion for our chiropractic mission. We will make the effort to care about our patients and their health, and to look after them better than any other doctor ever has, or ever will.

To make your recall procedures even more effective and well-received, I suggest you make a big deal about your special "recall service." Brag about it to your patients. Tell them about it long before they are ever in a position to be recalled. You should even list it as a special service of your practice in your practice brochure and other marketing tools you might be using.

Guidelines for Contacts

Never call the patient at work. The best time to call the patient at home is between 4:30 P.M. and 5:30 P.M. This is when the majority of individuals are arriving home from work, but before they are sitting down for their evening meal. Unfortunately, this is also the busiest time in most chiropractic offices. Therefore, whenever possible, it is wise to assign this task to someone other than the front desk CA.

The caller should speak only with the patient. Never leave a message either with another person or on an answering machine. (If another family member answers the phone, you may inquire as to when would be a good time to reach the patient.)

Should the CA encounter a patient who reveals that they are having continued problems, the CA should sympathize with them, and ask if the patient would like the doctor to call them.

The CA should always note the highlights of the conversation on the patient information card and initial it. This gives you a documented account of all follow-ups and attempted follow-ups with the patient, and may reveal a problem with the patient's chiropractic understanding. That may subsequently be dealt with on a follow-up visit.

Step 3-10: Efficient Scheduling and the Appointment Book System

The office appointment book is one of the most important tools used in any professional office. In fact, every other activity in the office revolves around the appointment schedule. Whether kept on the computer (electronic) or on the desk (printed) the proper size and usage of the appointment book will greatly assist in the development of your desired practice. Improper use, lack of disciplined scheduling procedures, or too small of an appointment book will just as surely prevent the realization of the practice of your dreams.

The biggest problem seen in most appointment books themselves is that they are simply too small. If you want your practice to continue to grow, you must continue to find larger appointment books. Strange as it may seem, I have actually consulted with doctors who cannot understand why their practice will not grow beyond a certain level, when their appointment book, in fact, does not have enough openings in the day to allow for the desired growth. It is difficult for the CA to book more patients than the appointment book has spaces.

Before you look at your appointment book, decide on how many patients you wish to see in any given day. Calculate the actual time you will spend with these patients. Do not forget the number of new patients and how much time each will take to process. How about reevaluations? Case reviews? Now, look carefully at your current appointment book. Count the spaces and time apportionment. Using this appointment book, is it physically possible for your CA to schedule the patients you want to see into this book? If not, get a bigger book. In fact, get a book that will allow for the scheduling of twice as many patients than you actually envision scheduling in a day. Remember, in all of nature vacuums are filled. Therefore, it is necessary for any growing practice, or a practice that wishes to grow, to be using a book that allows for a minimum of 50 to 100 percent more patient visits than the goal for daily patient visits.

A large appointment book is of little use, however, if the CA has no control over the scheduling process and does not book patients into specific, efficiently used blocks of time. Later we will discuss the benefits of block-booking patients. Before we do, again count the actual number of possible patients who can be seen in your book. Is there room for the growth you desire?

Earlier we discussed the importance of the forcing technique of proper scripting to guide the patient into the desired time for an appointment. The reason for this is that we want to block-book patients into specific areas of time that will allow specific procedures to be performed. For instance, by booking all regular adjustments into specific areas of time throughout the day, appropriate times may then be reserved for scheduling visits that may take longer, such as new patients, reevaluations, or case reviews. Block-booking patients is the key to efficiency in a chiropractic office. The CA must be trained in the proper concepts of block booking, the forcing technique, and the scripts necessary for such a procedure to be implemented.

Properly implemented, block-booking regular patient visits into four specific blocks of time—early and late morning, and early and late afternoon—leaves ample open time for reevaluations, re-consultations, and other activities that are vital in patient case management yet take more time to complete. Properly scheduled, these activities will never be missed or rescheduled because adequate time was not allowed.

Step 3-11: Charting Systems— Accurate and Quick

Proper recording of the patient's remarks and the procedures entered on a visit-by-visit basis is of the utmost value in protecting you from possible malpractice allegations, as well as enabling you to accurately produce a record of the patient's subjective response to your recommendations and care.

◆ Devise Systems for Success and Stability ◆

Good note-taking habits will enable you to accurately answer any questions that may be asked of you regarding your patient's care and their actual response to that care for years to come. Good note-taking, however, does not translate to large volumes of notes that slow you down and reinforce the presence or absence of symptoms to the patient. Unfortunately, in the proper caring for most patients, relief may be gradual and little change is reported on a visit-by-visit basis. Like watching children grow, the changes are incremental and often unnoticed over the limited time frame of one visit to another. Therefore, only pertinent notes should be recorded during the initial phase of relief care. More in-depth and sensible changes will be noted in the subjective portion of the reevaluation procedures, which will be performed in regular, but greater, intervals.

All progress notes and adjustment procedures should be documented on the patient information card so that on every visit you will have the patient's history at your fingertips, ready to be referred to. You should design a consistent way to record what adjustments were given—where and how. Often, this is totally dependent on the doctor's technique. In addition, efforts should be made to continually strive to reduce note taking while still maintaining the necessary information. Long, voluminous notes are not necessarily something to take pride in. Efficiency and effectiveness are.

Insurance Reporting

The insurance carrier will, at times, request copies of a patient's records, including all progress notes taken in the course of the patient's care. These requests usually indicate an attempt by the carrier to deny, or at best delay, benefits to the patient for prolonged care. To successfully limit the policyholder's benefits for chiropractic care, the carrier must determine that the patient is not being seen for either an illness or an injury, but merely for maintenance or wellness care.

Therefore, it is becoming increasingly important for you to efficiently document all of the patient's complaints on each office visit, as well as the patient's objective findings, on a regular basis. This record, along with the examination, x-ray, and case history findings will help to justify the need for continued care to third-party payers. Proper note taking will help ensure the patient's rights to insurance benefits and the patient's ability to continue to receive the long-term corrective and rehabilitative care most cases demand.

Progress Tracking

To record the patient's progress properly, during initial intensive or condition-based care, you must inquire as to the symptomatic status of the patient on each and every office visit and then record the patient's comments as briefly and succinctly as possible in the proper area of the patient information card. Often, this is neither as easy nor as simple as it sounds. (This may later be altered during the health or wellness phases of the patient's care.)

When you first encounter the patient and ask that tired old greeting, "How are you doing today?" the patient will often respond, "Good" or "Fine." If you find yourself falling into this pattern, you must remember to be aware that this phrase is usually a stock or conditioned answer rather than a true reflection of the patient's actual physical condition. Human nature being what it is, such stock answers must never be robotically recorded in the patient's progress notes. Instead, you must always question the patient further on the precise status of the patient's presenting condition.

Acquiring the necessary data may be easily accomplished by further questioning the patient about the general area of the original complaint, recent levels of activity, or specific types of situations or positions that the patient originally indicated would aggravate the condition. Clues to such information should have been gathered during the initial consultation and history.

In the same vein, never record the patient's remarks in one word, such as "good, bad, hurts, sore, etc." It will reflect poorly on your professionalism, competence, and may be quite damaging to both your reputation and the patient's care. This type of record-keeping falls far below the present-day standards demanded by today's courts, the insurance industry, and the rest of the professional community.

These remarks may cause others to construe such records to imply that the patient's condition may not have been serious enough to warrant your close attention, and, therefore, dismiss any pending insurance claims as meaningless or not clinically indicated.

Monitoring Patient Changes

When the patient begins to demonstrate improvements in his or her symptom complex, the records should always reflect exactly what has improved and to what extent. If the patient has worsened, the records must reflect that also. Quite often, patients will also report that he or she has not improved or the situation has even worsened. Often, these reports will imply that their care is not as effective as they anticipated, or that they are becoming discontented with their rate of response. Such might simply indicate a degree of misunderstanding of the resolution phases of their situation. When a patient reports a worsening condition or an exacerbation of their complaint, you should always attempt to question the patient further as to what may have transpired to aggravate the condition. More in-depth questioning and subsequent documentation of the actual mechanism that may have worsened or aggravated the patient's condition will take the responsibility for the worsening condition away from you, and document the necessity of continuing care.

Recording this exchange is important for three reasons. First, it may protect you from possible malpractice allegations should the patient claim the condition has worsened because of your care. Second, it may demonstrate to the insurance company that the patient has been reinjured, and the existence of a documented reinjury may help to justify any extended care that the patient may have required. Finally, if the patient fails to have obtained the expected results and becomes discouraged, you can quickly scan your annotations of the case and remind the patient of a previous incident that may have delayed recovery and prolonged the length of care beyond what you had originally prognosticated.

Expert Witness—Courtroom Testimony

In personal injury and workers' compensation claims, the value and necessity of complete progress notes are even more critical. If you practice long enough, it is almost assured that sooner or later you will actually be cross-examined in deposition or a court of law on matters regarding a patient's specific complaints, improvements, and services that were rendered on a specific date. Often, the office visit in question may have occurred several years earlier, and a competent attorney will quickly and easily discredit your testimony if proper notations have not been made at the time of service and if you attempt to testify based solely upon memory.

Patient Management During Corrective Care

When the patient has progressed through the symptomatic stage of care, and even though he or she is no longer expressing subjective complaints, proper questioning remains vitally important in the professional management of the case. In fact, proper questioning at this point becomes your most valuable tool in effective patient management.

Rather than asking the patient about symptomatology, the emphasis must shift from the patient's telling you how they feel, to your telling the patient about the progress being made. This is the stage of patient care where it is not only important for care to be justified for possible third party reimbursement, but for the patient as well.

Remember, most patients only go to a doctor when they are ill or in pain—for the relief of symptoms. After their symptoms have subsided, they will begin to question (either consciously or subconsciously) the need for continued care. The following procedure is designed to answer these questions before they are ever asked:

After two or three visits past the resolution of the patient's entrance complaints, you must *stop* inquiring about the patient's symptoms, and now begin to palpate the patient's spine (especially the area of the original complaint) to locate areas of soreness, edema, spastic muscles, and taut and tender fibers. Here especially, as patients move from the symptomatic phase of care into the corrective (asymptomatic) phase of care, the use of chiropractic instrumentation is vital in continued case management.

These areas must be quickly brought to the patient's attention, both subjectively and objectively. The patient must be made to understand that even though the area is essentially symptom free, that sub-symptomatic structural problems remain. These findings must then be recorded appropriately in the patient's progress notes. Such notations should describe the anatomical part involved, your findings in these areas (such as "right trapezius spasticity" or "pain and edema in left sacroiliac"), and the actual procedure that elicited positive responses.

By developing the habits of proper note-taking, you are documenting the patient's complaints, your objective findings, the specific adjustment rendered, and any extenuating circumstances. At the same time, you are also demonstrating your thoroughness, concern, and the patient's need for care. The few minutes necessary to do this properly will help protect you and your reputation, as well as the health and rights of your patient.

Key Points

- The creation and use of specific personalized office brochures can effectively transmit the vital information all patients should be given.
- The well-designed patient information card is the single most effective tool in managing your patients that can be incorporated into a chiropractic office.
- The most efficient means of communicating the services that were rendered, and the charges made on each visit and when the patient should return is by using a patient "service slip" at each visit.
- The use of case management plans and multiple appointment programs are powerful ways to build and add stability to the practice.
- The doctor's reinforcement of when and why to return, and the front desk's proper booking techniques, are the best way to prevent patients from leaving the office without a future appointment and drifting back to a subluxated life.
- The goal of the front desk should be that every patient who leaves the office has an appointment for a return visit, unless the doctor specifies otherwise.
- Once a patient has missed an appointment, the first 15 to 30 minutes are critical in contacting the patient and keeping him or her on schedule.
- Proper recalling, with the right scripts and attitude, helps to build goodwill toward your office and maintains a bond with past patients.
- If you want your practice to continue to grow, you must continue to find larger appointment books.
- Proper recording of the patient's remarks and the procedures entered on a visit-by-visit basis is of the utmost value in protecting you from possible malpractice allegations, as well as enabling you to accurately produce a record of the patient's subjective response to your recommendations and care.

Solution 4

Create Financial Policies to Grow Your Practice

The key to enjoying high collection ratios, patient compliance, and new patient referrals is to develop a comprehensive payment policy and fee structure that is well communicated and consistently administered. Such policies and fees will effectively promote the development and expansion of your practice.

The establishment of clear and reasonable financial procedures greatly simplifies what could otherwise be a frustrating aspect of office management. For obvious reasons, collections are the most important nonclinical aspect of office management. Successfully managed and used, effective collection procedures must provide a high ratio of collections vs. services while maintaining good patient relations.

To avoid confusion and "buck-passing" there must be one person in the office who is both designated and highly trained to handle all financial arrangements with the patient. In every case, I recommend this person *not* be the doctor. Whenever the doctor gets involved with financial arrangements, one thing always happens—accounts receivable go up.

The most obvious person to be responsible for initial implementation of the financial policies with each patient should be the person who is charged with executing the financial arrangement over the course of the patient's care. Because it is the CA's responsibility to ultimately enforce the collection procedures and agreements, it is only natural that he or she be the one making the initial arrangements within the guidelines of set policies and established procedures. This arrangement prevents patients from pitting one staff member against the other and claiming that different arrangements were made when collection time is at hand.

It is essential that the CA be well versed in each of the various financial policies, and comfortable with them. It is more important that he or she present them to every new patient in a clear and concise manner, as well as answer all questions with confidence and certainty. If the CA has done the job of initially befriending the new patient, and gaining their confidence on the first visit, then, by the second visit, he or she should be the person the patient is most at ease with discussing such issues as finances and then making the appropriate commitments. Remember, while the doctor is responsible for designing and overseeing the collection policies and procedures, the doctor never talks money with the patient. And all discussion and arrangements about payment and payment options stops with the office policy regarding each conceivable situation.

Determining Patient/Payment Type

Knowing how to proceed with a new patient financially is important in preparing paperwork and making collections for the first visit. The patient financial options form will immediately answer this question. I recommend that this form be placed on the clipboard with the initial new patient forms. It effectively gives the patient early information on established financial policies while notifying the CA as to how to proceed. It is important that the patients receive, read, understand, complete, and sign this form before seeing the doctor. It is, without a doubt, the first step in gaining control of the financial dealings with the patient. And, it sets the stage for the enactment of every other financial policy that will be instituted in your practice.

Step 4-1: Give the Cash Patient Financial Options

The cash patient may present in one of three variations. The patient may have no major medical insurance coverage. The patient who has major medical insurance coverage, but does not wish to use it, wishes to self-file, or refuses to assign the benefits of the policy to the doctor. Or, depending on the type of practice, it may be a personal injury patient.

Patient Financial Options

Although most offices may expect the cash patient to pay at the time service is rendered, most patients with problems that require extended initial intensive or corrective care may be unable to budget enough for such care. For the practice to demand payment in full on each visit only serves to disqualify many uninsured patients from the practice, withholding help from those who may need chiropractic care the most. No patient should ever be denied chiropractic care based on his or her ability to pay. Instead, creative options should be developed and the office should have a menu of payment options available to the cash patient.

Preset policies that allow patients to receive needed care will not only benefit the patient, but also your practice and your reputation. If, however, financial arrangements are made, preset and written policies describing acceptable arrangements are an absolute necessity for the CA to function effectively. In addition to policy, effective collection procedures and scripts are vital to reducing stress and getting the results wanted.

The proper procedures for making financial arrangements with cash patients include having a frank, private discussion with every patient as to the anticipated cost of care, presenting various *acceptable* methods of payment, and setting an agreeable day or date for payment.

In addition, to prevent future problems from arising, a brief discussion of the office's policy for failure to keep agreed-upon arrangements should be reviewed with the patient as well. Acquiring both a verbal and written commitment from the patient to make a specified, uninterrupted schedule of payments and for the patient to agree to pay off all outstanding balances in full if care should be discontinued prematurely, will help prevent patient attrition.

Possible Arrangements for the Cash Patient

Clearly, the more and varied payment arrangement possibilities the office can present, the more likely the patient will be able to afford to receive the necessary care. In addition, devising and providing sufficient payment plans for cash patients gives the impression that the office is reasonable, concerned, and willing to help the patient. Individual offices can design their own options for payment that are in line with their attitudes and state laws. Examples of such payment options include:

1. Payment in full at the beginning of care for a certain percentage discount;
2. Allowing the patient to pay in full at the end of each week rather than at each visit;
3. Weekly payments averaging the total anticipated care over a several-week or -month period;
4. Credit card authorization to charge payment at the end of each week. (Maybe with a slight discount.)

The above are simply ideas; use your imagination and develop arrangements that may fit with your practice and your beliefs. Above all, acceptable payment arrangements should be designed to make it easy for the cash-paying patient to stay, pay, and get well. Every effort should be made to have the vast majority of the cost of services paid by the end of the patient's period of initial intensive care. If, however, the practice has a large degree of wellness carry-over, and, in the judgment of both you and your CA, the patient is sincere, payments may be stretched out past initial intensive care and into the first few months of wellness care.

Collection Procedures for Cash Patients

Once a fair, mutually agreed-upon financial arrangement has been made, it is up to the staff to make the agreed-upon collections at the proper time. Failure of the staff to collect from the patient or failure to enforce the agreed-upon arrangements hurts both the patient and the practice.

♦ Devise Systems for Success and Stability ♦

Documented studies from the dental profession have shown that patients who are in arrears to their doctor cannot *allow* themselves to experience good results. ("Why should I pay? That doctor didn't help me" is the subliminal message that seems to develop when an overdue bill is owed.) We also know that patients who are behind in their payments or owe the doctor money will naturally tend to avoid the doctor and not receive needed care. Appointments are more likely to be either broken or missed. What a disservice to the patient.

We also know that patients who are delinquent in payments tend to resent the doctor and seldom refer (or worse, refer similar patients). Then, when collection proceedings are instituted, the possibilities of malpractice allegations against the doctor increase proportionally.

For these reasons, it is important that collections proceed as agreed upon. All arrangements with the patients should be written on the patient's ledger card or noted on the office computer, and collections made as a routine (and important) aspect of the CA's job.

Step 4-2: Develop Effective Procedures and Reasonable Policies for the Insured Patient

Knowing how to proceed with a new patient (especially a patient with group major medical coverage) on a financial basis is important in preparing paperwork, obtaining necessary information, and knowing what to collect on the first visit and thereafter. The "patient financial options form" (see page 147) will immediately tell the CA how to proceed. When patients indicate they believe they have insurance coverage and will comply with the "rules of engagement," it becomes essential for the CA to initiate the procedures necessary to handle this patient service effectively.

Verifying Coverage

The first activity to be embarked upon by the CA is to verify that the patient does indeed have insurance coverage, and the extent of that coverage. Although many patients do have group or personal health coverage, today's policies are so varied in their insurance benefits that specific coverage should never be taken for granted. For this reason, it is essential that the CA or the business manager contact the insurance carrier immediately to determine policy coverage, amounts, and limitations.

After the new patient completes the new patient induction forms, the CA should immediately note if the patient has checked the "cash option" or the "insurance option" on the patient financial options form. If "insurance" was checked, the CA should immediately ask the patient for their insurance card.

From the card, the CA can then obtain the insured patient's name, policy numbers, address, and phone number of the insurance company. A photocopy of the card may be taken at this time. (Minimally, all information on the card should be written down.)

Remember...any patient who cannot produce an insurance card will be considered a cash patient until one is produced and coverage verified.

Once the patient has been taken back for new patient processing, the CA should immediately call the insurance company and attempt to verify the limits of coverage. The insurance verification worksheet should be used to obtain all the needed information. Remember, in most cases, the insurance representative is providing this information as a courtesy and as such, the CA must be polite and grateful. The script may go something like this:

CA: "Hello. This is Carol from Dr. Meyer's office. I would like to verify coverage on one of your policyholders. Could you tell me what the deductible and coinsurance are on this policy? Has the deductible been met? Are there any limitations or maximum limits on covered services?"

Once the worksheet has been completed and the patient's insurance card copied onto the reverse side of the worksheet, the CA should have all of the information needed to proceed with making the appropriate collections for the first visit.

Discussion of First Day's Fees

Many offices struggle with the dilemma of how to approach the subject of the first day's fees with the patient. Unfortunately, when a patient calls and expresses a concern over the amount of the first day's fees, unless you have one, set rate for fees, the CA will not be able to give the patient one specific price. Obviously, the CA (nor the doctor)

◆ Create Financial Policies to Grow Your Practice ◆

Insurance Verification
(Worksheet)

☐ Group Insurance   ☐ Worker's Compensation   ☐ Medicare
☐ Personal Injury   ☐ Other:_____   ☐ Medicaid

Patient's Name:_____   Date:_____
Insured:_____   Phone:_____
Relation To Insured: ☐ Self   ☐ Spouse   ☐ Child   Other:_____
Insured's Employer:_____   Phone:_____

GROUP INSURANCE

Name of Insurance Company:_____   Phone:_____
Insurance Contact:_____   Extension #:_____
     Is there coverage for chiropractic care?............................... ☐ Yes   ☐ No
     What are the policy limits or restrictions:............................... _____
     What is the deductible: .... $_____
     Has deductible been met for year?...................................... ☐ Yes   ☐ No
     What is coverage after deductible?...................................... _____ / _____
     When is deductible due?..
     Are diagnostics applied to deductible?................................. ☐ Yes   ☐ No
     Does this policy cover:
         X-rays & Examination... ☐ Yes   ☐ No
         Chiropractic adjustments:.. ☐ Yes   ☐ No
         Physical therapy:... ☐ Yes   ☐ No
         Orthopedic supports:... ☐ Yes   ☐ No
     Will your company honor an "Assignment of Benefits"?............. ☐ Yes   ☐ No

WORKER'S COMPENSATION

Employer:_____   Phone:_____
Employer contact:_____   Ext: _____
Has injury been reported?... ☐ Yes   ☐ No

COPY
Front of Insurance Card

COPY
Back of Insurance Card

Sample Form: **Insurance Verification Worksheet**

will not know what level new patient exam or which x-ray studies will be indicated. Hence, the CA will usually not be able to accurately quote a first visit cost. This will prove frustrating for the prospective patient as well as the staff. And, while there may not be one absolutely perfect way to handle every prospective patient caller, the following procedure will usually satisfy the *majority* of new patients with such concerns.

Like all financial matters, it is important to always address the subject of fees and their payment in as open and up-front a manner as possible. When the patient inquires as to the first visit fees, the CA should respond with the concept that every patient is different, requiring different levels of service. The CA should invite the patient to make an appointment to discuss their concerns with the doctor, after which the doctor will have an idea as to the indicated procedures in the case and can give an educated estimate. The proper way to do so is quite simple, but it requires good communication between the CA and the doctor. Should the patient, at any point express a concern about the first day's costs, the CA must communicate this to the doctor prior to the new patient consultation. Then, after the consultation, when the doctor has a better idea as to the level of examination and x-rays that are indicated, the doctor will mark the service slip appropriately, and then say to the patient:

> **Doctor:** "Mrs. Jones, Carol noted that you had asked about fees for this visit. So before we go any further, let me give you an idea as to what we will need to do today.
>
> "First, the primary purpose of today's visit it to determine the real nature of your health concerns. Based on what you have told me, we should not take this concern lightly. Therefore, I am going to recommend that we do an intermediate new patient examination. This will give me a good idea as to the nature of this situation. A set of full spine pictures are indicated so that we can see the true, underlying cause of your problems.
>
> "As you may know, I have a reputation of being thorough and complete. That is because I would rather not have you as a patient at all, than to accept you as a patient and not do everything necessary to give you my the best care possible.

"Now, I am not allowed to discuss fees with my patients, because I usually give the wrong answer...so, if you would like, I can have Carol come in and review the fees for these services, and then, if everything is acceptable to you we will get started. Fair enough?"

It is important the CA remains alert and close to the door should the doctor need a fee review with the patient. If at all possible, the doctor may simply open the door at the beginning of the above script as a signal for the CA to enter. In many cases, once the patient accepts the first day's fees, the CA may actually proceed with gathering much of the objective findings in the examination prior to the doctor's return.

Collection of First Day Fees

If the patient has health insurance that you believe (from previous experience with the carrier) will cover the services in your office, your first day's collection procedures should be minimal. It is important, however, that the patient be made aware of the charges for the first visit and that nothing about your procedures appears secretive or hidden. Therefore, after the initial visit has been completed, the front desk CA should review all charges for the first visit with the patient and attempt to collect those fees.

Therefore, when the new patient is returned to the front desk, the CA should place the fee slip on the counter in front of the patient, point to the different services that were given, and say:

> *CA:* "Mrs. Jones, today the doctor performed an in-depth consultation and health history for which there was no charge. The chiropractic examination was $75, and the x-rays were $150. That comes to $225 for today. Will that be cash, check, or credit card?"

If the patient asks about insurance coverage for these fees, rather than trying to discuss the details at this time, the CA should merely state:

> *CA:* "I will call your insurance company this afternoon to check your coverage and review it with you tomorrow."

If the new patient does not have insurance coverage (or you have a good idea that the policy does not cover their services), you should make the same effort to collect as above.

However, if the patient hesitates or can only make a partial payment, the staff should be gracious, but never state that it is "okay" or that it is "no problem." Instead, the CA should inform the patient that they "understand" the situation, and that arrangements will be made on the next visit.

CA: "I understand, Mrs. Jones; we'll set up some arrangements tomorrow."

The most important point to remember is that (if everything was done correctly) the patient has just enjoyed a wonderful experience in your office. They have met a warm and caring staff, and received a thorough consultation and comprehensive examination by a doctor who is warm, compassionate, and caring. The front desk, within view of other patients, is *not* the time to undo the goodwill that was developed throughout the first visit by utilizing heavy-handed collection techniques.

When the patient leaves the office after the first visit, you, your staff, and all of your procedures should have worked collectively to make certain that patient is on "cloud nine." You want them to be excited about their first experience in your office and confident that they have absolutely found the right doctor and the right practice for them and their family. If every procedure was explained and the fees were handled in an open, up-front, and professional manner, the new patient should not be confused or fretting about the issue of money at this time. Except for the patient who expressed a concern about the initial charges, any possible problems with making financial arrangements or pursuing collections are more easily made on the second visit, after the case review, and behind closed doors.

Whatever the policies for collecting the first day's charges, both the doctor and the CA must remember that the first day collection tactics should never be so heavy-handed or rigid as to dampen the excitement and enthusiasm that were generated during the patient's first visit experience.

Step 4-3: Insurance/Co-Payment Determination for Painless Collections

As the second visit draws near, and the doctor makes the determination as to the long-term recommendations that will be given the patient, the CA must begin to prepare a financial report in which he or she will discuss the costs and various payment options for attaining such care.

The CA cannot determine the actual amount of weekly payments the patient will make until the doctor completes the patient information card and returns it with the recommended level of care marked. (See recommendations and MAP scheduling.) Once this has been completed, the CA can then simply plug in the appropriate numbers in the insurance co-payment determination worksheet (see page 216) according to the recommended level of care the patient will require.

The insurance co-payment determination worksheet factors in the first visit charges,
The costs of the recommended care, the level of the patient's coinsurance, the deductible amount, and the number of payments following charges for the patient. Weighing these factors will allow the CA to determine the average weekly payment necessary to satisfy all of the various contingencies. It should be mentioned that the formula provided should be followed exactly as it appears on the worksheet, regardless of whether the patient's deductible has been met or not.

Immediately following the first visit, the doctor should complete the first section. Each blank space represents one week of the first three months that the patient may require care. Here the doctor writes his recommendations as to number of visits each week for the first 90 days.

With this information, the CA who handles the financial arrangements can then calculate the total fees for the case for the first 90 days. Accurately doing so then allows the total cost of the case to be calculated to a weekly payment for the insured patient. Using the formula on the worksheet, the amount of weekly payments should seem almost ridiculously low to the patient.

Financial Review (Second Visit)

On the patient's next visit the doctor will present their case report, detailing the three primary objectives of care and the actual recommendations necessary to achieve the desired objectives. Following the case report, the patient will have a working knowledge of their situation, the promises of effective chiropractic care, and the doctor's recommendations for achieving the agreed-upon objectives.

With the proper case report, the doctor will get a firm commitment from the patient to follow through with the recommended care, and make absolutely certain that the patient understands the totality of the frequency and duration of care. If the patient asks about fees and payment at that time, the doctor will always defer to the CA who will present the financial review immediately following the case report. If the doctor has delivered a good case report and the patient thoroughly understands every aspect of it, a high percentage of the patients will accept the recommended objectives and care. The CA's financial review should then be a quick and easy task.

Most critical to the accomplishment of making specific financial arrangements by the CA, is that the doctor has prepared the patient successfully. Once the doctor has determined that the patient fully accepts the case report and case recommendations, the doctor should wrap up the case review by asking the patient to remain seated while the CA comes into the office to review the financial aspects of care.

Doctor: "Mrs. Jones, is there anything I didn't fully explain to you? Or do you have any other questions? If not, I would like you to remain seated while Carol comes in and gives you the good news about your insurance. I will see you in the adjusting room in a couple of minutes, and we will get started on correcting the cause of your nerve interference."

CA: "Mrs. Jones, I confirmed your insurance coverage yesterday with your insurance company, and they will cover most, but not all, of your care in our office. Based on your coverage, and what the doctor has recommended, I have averaged the cost to you over the next (insert number) weeks. Your approximate amount would be $ (insert number) at the end of each week. Then, by the time your recommended care is completed, your portion should be all caught up.

"Do you have any problems with this amount? If not, will it be convenient to pay it on your last visit of each week?"

◆ Create Financial Policies to Grow Your Practice ◆

Patient Agreement
Regarding Non-Insurance Payment Option

We are happy to offer you several choices of payment for the program of care you are about to receive in our office. As an alternative to collecting fees at each visit, we have developed these options to streamline your payments and to remove any financial obstacles. Our intent is to make it both convenient and less costly for you to receive the care that you need.

RECOMMENDED CARE: _____ VISITS

ANTICIPATED TIME _____ WEEKS

ESTIMATED INVESTMENT $_____

☐ Payment In full at beginning of care.
  (15% Discount — Save $_____)

☐ Credit card authorization (to charge balance of account at end of week.)
  (10% Discount - Save $_____)

☐ Weekly Payment Average Plan:
  _____ post-dated checks in the amount of $_____.
  (5% Discount—Save $_____)

☐ Payment in full after each visit.

PATIENT AGREEMENT

In selecting the above payment option, I agree:

1. To make uninterrupted payments based on the option that I have selected until my account balance reaches zero.
2. That (unless other arrangements are made) no further care shall be rendered should any payment become seven (7) days past due.
3. That if I discontinue care for any reason (other than discharge by doctor) all outstanding balances shall immediately become due and payable.
4. That if I have pre-paid for my care, and if for any reason I must discontinue care, all unused portions of the advance payment will be returned, less any discount applied.

The above options and all costs associated with my care in this office have been thoroughly explained to me. I wish to participation in this plan of payment for the professional services that I will receive.

_____   _____
Signature of Patient or Guardian   *Date*

Sample Form: **Patient Agreement**

In addition to the agreement for timely and preset payments, the CA must also have the patient sign the "directive for disbursement" form (assignment). The proper timing is to present this form after arrangements have been made. Such an order to the insurance company is now understandable and reasonable to the patient. This directive will be vital in protecting the practice and to ensure that the insurance benefits are sent to the practice—not the patient.

Special Note

The effectiveness of the CA in designing and presenting the fee and payment policies and procedures is completely dependent on the relationship that he or she has developed with the new patient. Most critical, however, is the doctor's ability to perform a thorough consultation and examination and then present an effective case review with strong, objective-based recommendations.

Step 4-4: Play the Third-Party Pay and Personal-Injury Game by Your Rules

Although many doctors accept personal injury cases, I have found that, unless handled properly, with well-designed, strictly enforced policies, such cases often become a source of stress to the staff and lost income to the doctor. Yes, it is true these patients need care, and for us to refuse to care for these types of patients may be inhumane. Yet, I maintain that you can care appropriately for the patient, and yet effectively remove yourself from the third-party "Bermuda Triangle."

The secret is to design written and enforceable policies that will allow these patients to come under your care, according to your rules. The biggest mistake many doctors make is to defer the establishment of payment policies in these cases to the patient, the insurance adjuster, or worse, the attorney. The attitude I recommend is that you remain in control. Remember that in your office it is your game and your rules. If you run into adjustors, attorneys, and patients who do not want to play by the rules, then they may have to sit out the game.

It has been my experience that, with personal injury patients, it is difficult to achieve good results. More than not, their ultimate financial settlement levels are based upon the amount of care they receive or the size of the bills they amass. Attorneys routinely advise their clients of this, and, as a result, patients are too often less than motivated to allow themselves to get well.

Anyone who has had the experience of handling personal injury patients will tell you that such cases always require additional time in documentation and paperwork. With personal injury patients, the doctor will spend an inordinate amount of time preparing reports to attorneys and insurance companies. Unfortunately, the amount charged for depositions and courtroom appearances, and the amount that attorneys are willing to pay are seldom equal to the income that can be derived from staying in the office and caring for "regular" patients. Worst of all, the secondary activities associated with caring for personal injury patients will certainly detract from your energy and your time spent with other patients or in fulfilling your personal and practice mission.

Considering all of the additional time and effort expended in managing these cases, and the fact that most doctors often do not see any payment for their services for several years, one has to wonder why any chiropractor would ever accept personal injury cases.

Much of the frustration encountered with personal injury cases can be avoided if it is understood that these cases usually fall into two distinct categories. The first comprises patients who want to use the doctor and his or her expertise to build their case. These patients are only interested in the financial gain represented by an imminent insurance or legal settlement. The second group consists of those patients who are truly sincere about getting well. Unfortunately, it is initially difficult to tell the difference between the two. With either group, most personal injury patients enter your practice with the assumption that some other party is responsible for payment of their care, and that it is *your* responsibility to care for them and, not only to wait for payment, but to act as their agent in securing that payment.

This erroneous concept must be dealt with immediately before you can develop a positive doctor-patient relationship and successfully handle this case on a clinical and business level. The patient must know they are contracting with you for their services and that you expect payment in full, on a timely basis, regardless of any settlement with a third party. In addition, you must make it clear that you and your practice are not and will not become an interested party in the outcome of any legal settlement. I encourage you to never want or need a patient so badly that you are not prepared to refer an uncooperative personal injury patient to another provider. No matter what, the patient must always be accepted on your terms based on predetermined and written policies. Exceptions to this policy are always problems in both the long- and short-term and should never be undertaken.

In most circumstances, the CA will be the first to become aware of this type of patient. The patient financial options form will identify these patients at the outset since there is no option available for these types of cases. In these situations, the patient will either inform the CA that a third party will be responsible for paying the doctor, or the patient will not know how to complete the form. As soon as the CA realizes the new patient wants the practice to "carry" their account, established (written) financial policies must be reviewed and specific financial arrangements must be made *before* the patient sees the doctor for the initial consultation and exam. Dealing with the situation afterward is usually much more difficult and always less effective.

Therefore, when a personal injury case enters the office, as with any new patient, the CA should welcome them and request all of the appropriate paperwork be completed. Once the patient has finished their new patient induction forms, the CA should take the patient to the consultation room and explain the practice's financial and payment policies regarding personal injury case management.

Optimally, the patient should be accepted as a regular cash or major medically insured patient. All financial agreements must be explained, agreed to, and signed with all of the proper arrangements agreed upon. The only way that insurance may be accepted is if the patient obtains a written agreement with the liable insurance company to pay all charges as submitted on a monthly basis. The financial arrangement and agreement form gives the personal patient a choice of how to handle their account in your office. Providing a menu of acceptable payment arrangements lets the patient feel you are not being dictatorial in your approach and that your staff is willing to work out an agreement for the necessary care. It should be presented in the following way:

CA: "Mrs. Jones, before the doctor comes in, I would like to review with you the practice policy for handling the financial aspects of personal injury cases such as yours.

"It is this practice's policy not to accept assignment on these types of cases. That simply means that we are prohibited from carrying your balance and waiting for you to settle with the liable insurance company for your bill to be paid in our office.

"This is because most insurance companies will not pay for your care until you sign off of this claim. Depending on the case, that may take months or even years—especially if an attorney becomes involved.

"Therefore, I am required to make specific financial arrangements with the patient, not their insurance company or their attorney.

"Of course, the doctor will prepare any reports that your insurance company or your attorney may request, and cooperate with them so that you may successfully make settlement, but you will be financially responsible for all of your care in our office and we will not look to a third party to pay your bill.

"We can, however, make financial arrangements for your care if necessary. Those arrangements include:

Note: The following examples are simply ideas of various arrangements that may be entered into with PI patients. They may not be appropriate for your practice or even consistent with the laws of the state in which you practice. I suggest you use your imagination and brainstorm these and other arrangements that will suit your practice and local laws.

1. You may make payment in full at the beginning of care and receive a 10 percent discount for the care the doctor has recommended.
2. You may pay as you go. In many cases, you can then take your receipts to the insurance company and they will reimburse you right away.
3. You may leave a credit card imprint, then you will not have to pay until the end of the month.
4. You may average your recommended care into three equal payments and leave three post-dated checks.

5. You may assign your major medical benefits to this office and we will bill your care to your major medical carrier; then you would only pay your deductible and coinsurance."

If You Do Accept Assignment

If the patient indicates a strong desire not to pay for the services, and you wish to make an exception (not recommended), assignment should be accepted only in the following manner:

> **CA:** "If you prefer not to handle your account in this manner, we do have two choices that are acceptable: (1) The office may accept assignment *if* your insurance company agrees to pay all charges as submitted on a monthly basis. To do this, you must ask them to complete this form and return it to us. When we receive the form back, we can begin care.
>
> "And (2), you can sign this assignment of benefits form, and instruct your attorney to sign an attorney lien form. This promises that your account will be paid to our office at settlement. However, even with both forms signed, we still require the patient to make uninterrupted weekly payments of $35 until final payment/settlement has been received.
>
> "Regardless of when your settlement may occur, we require that you promise to make full payment of all outstanding balances within 30 days after your dismissal from active care."

Although these provisions are certainly not preferable to the patient's keeping their account current, they will go a long way in protecting your fee and ultimately improving your chances of receiving payment.

In all honesty, you will find that most insurance carriers will refuse option one, especially should an attorney be (or become) involved. As liberal as it is, some patients will even refuse the second option. These people are, in fact, telling you that they have no desire to take responsibility for their own care and probably have no respect for you or your time and services. I suggest at this point, the CA politely inform the patient that these are the only two acceptable choices and that perhaps the patient would like to discuss the choices with a spouse or attorney and call back.

Create Financial Policies to Grow Your Practice

Directive For Disbursement
"Assignment of Insurance Benefits"

By this instrument, I authorize, instruct, and order any insurance company obligated by contractual agreement to reimburse me for allowable professional or medical services to make direct payment to:

_____
_____
_____

This payment shall be credited by the provider directly to my account, and I have agreed to pay (in a current manner) the balance of all charges for professional services over and above the insurance payment.

I also authorize the release of any information pertinent to my case to any insurance company, claims adjuster, or attorney involved in this case.

THIS IS A DIRECT ASSIGNMENT OF ALL BENEFITS TO THIS HEALTHCARE PROVIDER.

_____   _____
Signature of Policy Holder   Witness

_____   _____
Signature of Claimant   Date

A PHOTOCOPY OF THIS DOCUMENT SHALL BE AS VALID AS THE ORIGINAL

Sample Form: **Directive for Disbursement**

Remember, if your dream practice is a wellness or family-type practice, the personal injury patient is a patient who will consume much of your time and energy in dealing with their pain, documentation, reports, depositions, and court appearances. With all the time and effort that will be expended, you should not have to wait for your payment. If this patient does not wish to abide by the established office policies, you and your staff must hold true to the policies that you have implemented and refer the patient to another doctor. After almost 30 years of practicing, I still maintain that the loss of this type of patient, if they do not want to play by your rules, should not be lamented.

Personal Injury Financial Options

If the insurance company agrees to pay all charges as submitted on a monthly basis, your policy should be that the liable insurance company must complete a lien promising to pay all charges that the patient incurs on a monthly basis (whether or not an attorney is involved). Only when the form is returned, will care be rendered without patient payment.

In addition, the patient must sign the "directive to pay doctor" (assignment of benefits) form and the patient's attorney must sign the form as well. To improve patient compliance and to assist in offsetting the costs of care, the personal injury patient should be required to make uninterrupted monthly payments of $35 until final payment/settlement has been received and the patient further agrees to make full payment of all outstanding balances within 30 days after dismissal from active care.

Step 4-5: Develop Effective and Efficient Insurance Reporting Procedures

Whether you purposefully design an insurance-based practice, a cash practice, or a combination practice, patients will always ask that you reply to the myriad of various insurance questionnaires that their carriers will send to them. To simply refuse will lead to disgruntled patients and frequent premature patient attrition. To gladly accept and complete these forms will rob you of coveted patient time and distract from your true mission as a dedicated chiropractor. Most cases of doctor burnout we have witnessed have come from fatigue and frustration over these types of activities. As a response to these situations, we recommend instituting the following ways to reduce, streamline, or eliminate these frustrating demands on our time.

Ask Your Patient to Report to Their Insurer

Quite often, you will be asked by the patient or the patient's insurance carrier to justify care to a patient who may be considered to be in the "wellness phase" of care. And, while we may explain to the patient that they are not being seen for a specific diagnosed problem, rather to maintain their health, they will still expect insurance reimbursement. Understandably, after months or even years of patients submitting claims to their carrier, that carrier may appropriately question the care rendered. The same is true for the patient who comes in for frequent symptomatic exacerbations and then files his or her own insurance. Because these are often the lifelong patients upon which the practice is built, the doctor and the CA often feel obliged to assist this coveted patient and must expend both time and energy on these activities if for no other reason, than to keep this patient happy.

Such activities can be gently and significantly reduced by employing the preemptive procedure of giving the patient a "notice to insurance carrier" form to be filled out and sent to the insurer (by the patient) along with the patient's insurance claim form or super bill/service slip.

This form will answer the claim reviewer's questions before they are asked and it will eliminate the need for the doctor and staff to become involved in more paperwork and nonpatient care activities. Should the carrier deny the patient's claim and the patient subsequently asks the doctor or staff to submit further information, they may simply be told that they (the patient) have already given the insurer the same information that you could supply. Therefore, the doctor can then politely remove him- or herself from the "insurance-patient-provider triangle" by simply suggesting the insurance company be consulted directly by the patient. At this point, you may also provide the patient with the telephone number and address of their state's insurance commissioner's office. The patient may then contact the state agency and request their assistance with the matter.

Notice To Insurance Carrier

PLEASE BE ADVISED . . .

On ___/___/___ , I specifically sought care for the following complaint (s):

DEGREE   AREA OF COMPLAINT

☐ Mild: _____   ☐
Moderate: _____
    ☐ Severe: _____

These symptoms first appeared on: ___/___/___

These complaints were caused or worsened by:

CAUSE	DESCRIPTION	DATE
☐ Over-activity	_____	___/___/___
☐ Illness:	_____	___/___/___
☐ Injury:	_____	___/___/___
☐ Other:	_____	___/___/___
☐ Unknown:	_____	___/___/___

Since their onset, my symptoms have been:

☐ Improving   ☐ Unchanged   ☐ Getting Worse

PLEASE NOTE:

THIS CARE WAS NEITHER ROUTINE NOR MAINTENANCE.
Professional care was directed specifically toward the resolution
of the above complaint.

The benefits for this claim have **NOT** been assigned to the doctor.

Patient: _____
Insured: _____
Policy Number: _____
Employer: _____
    Signature: _____   ___/___/___

Attached are my insurance claim form and the attending doctor's statement.

Sample Form: **Notice to Insurance Carrier**

The notice to insurance carrier form should be given to the appropriate patient following each visit. As the form is given, the CA must provide instructions to the patient to complete it, and to submit it along with their claim to their insurer.

Response to Report Request

Too often, attorneys, insurance carriers, and yes, even patients attempt to pirate the doctor's time and energies away from the practice and family by requiring endless reports and redundant information submittals. Remember, these individuals are often paid by the hour themselves, so they have no concept of the value of a doctor's time as it relates to productivity. If providing attorney and insurance reports is a necessary aspect of your type of practice, at least you should be paid (and paid well) for your time. The most important factor that you, as a doctor, must remember is how valuable your time and knowledge actually is. Moreover, you must consider the income that you would be enjoying if you were using this time seeing patients instead of writing reports. With this in mind, it might be helpful to compute your actual gross income per hour and then charge accordingly.

Whenever a request for a report comes to the office there must be a system and procedure in place for dealing with it as well. When a request for a report is received, the CA should immediately send a statement for the report to the insurance company. On the statement, the requesting party should be advised that the request has been received but no action will be taken on the request until payment is received. (At times, it may be advantageous to copy this statement to the patient as well.) The information request should then be placed in a designated location with a copy of the statement attached. There it will remain with no further action taken until payment is received. When payment is received for the requested report, the CA will then place the request, the check, and the patient's full file on the doctor's desk for processing. The request should not be given to the doctor until payment is made. At the same time, the doctor should be disciplined to not cash the check until the report is completed and mailed.

If, during the time that the statement has been sent and payment received, the patient questions if the report has been completed and sent, the CA may simply tell the patient that the requesting party has

Statement For Doctor's Report

To: _____   Remit To:

Date: _____   _____

Re: Patient: _____   _____

ID #: _____   _____

Group/Employer: _____   _____

We have received your request for:
- ☐ Review of Records & Completion of Brief Report Form.
- ☐ Review of Records & Completion of Detailed Report
- ☐ Review of Records & Completion of Comprehensive Narrative Report.
- ☐ Special Report (Assessment, Treatment Plan, or Impairment Rating)
- ☐ Transmittal of Records.
- ☐ Other: _____

As you know, this information is more extensive and comprehensive than is usually required in quired in processing a standard health insurance claim. To properly respond to such a request places a burden on the doctor and increases the clerical overhead of a professional practice. Obviously, such undertakings result in additional expenses, which, in the end, contribute to the rising costs of healthcare for everyone.

In attempting to contain the costs of healthcare for our patients (and their insurers) we are diligently striving to keep our professional fees as low and as stable as possible. We believe that it would be unfair to allow our professional fees to escalate for <u>all</u> patients in order for us to recover the costs incurred by providing only a <u>few</u> insurance carriers with such comprehensive and in-depth information.

Therefore, we require the remittance of a fee of $____ prior to this office committing the time and resources necessary to prepare the report that you have requested.

If it is not the policy of your company to reimburse providers for their time and efforts in these matters, we ask that you make provisions with your policyholder to remit the above fee. Upon receiving payment, we will immediately undertake to provide you with the supplementary information that you have requested.

WE WILL NOT BILL OUR PATIENT FOR THIS FEE

Sample Form: **Statement for Doctor's Report**

been sent a statement for the doctor's time, but payment has not been received yet. The CA may encourage the patient to contact the person requesting the information and inquire as to the status of the pending payment. To expedite the process, the CA may give the patient the opportunity to pay for the services if they wish.

Eventually, the realization will come to the patient that third-party payers are not always as interested in the information they are requesting as they are in using stalling techniques to avoid paying their policyholder's claims, while earning interest on that same money. The above procedure is effective and efficient, but only when it is the patient, not the doctor, who is waiting for payment. Proper implementation of the systems and solutions presented in this book should prevent this situation from occurring.

Patient Response to Insurance Review

The following letter is useful in helping the patient take responsibility for dealing with a contrary insurance company. Unfair as it may be, whenever an insurance company does not pay for the services the patient thinks they should, the doctor ends up in the middle, and quite often is blamed for the lack of payment. In many situations, the innocent doctor becomes the bad guy if he tries to collect from the patient for services the insurer will not pay.

To combat this situation and help the patient comprehend the possible unfair and uncooperative tactics of their insurance carrier, the patient must be brought into a partnership with the doctor. This letter actually enlists the partnership of the patient in dealing with the insurance carrier. When the patient spends the time and energy writing a letter, that individual knows how much time and effort is involved for you, as well as how unfair and uncooperative the carrier may be.

This letter should be sent to any patient whenever a request for information or the initiation of a review is made. The CA should send this letter to the patient, and the doctor should not even begin the patient's report until the patient returns the requested letter. Quite often, when confronted with having to make an effort to do some of the work, the patient will decide the insurance payment simply is not worth it—thus leaving you and your staff off the hook.

Dear Patient:

Your insurance carrier, **XYZ Insurance Company**, is reviewing the claim that you submitted for the care that you received in this office. As such, they have requested a report by the doctor as well as a substantial amount of documentation pertaining to your health history, complaints, our findings in your case, the care that you have received, as well as any anticipated future care.

While the report from our office will be quite exhaustive, it is important that you also submit a letter to them. We have found that such a letter from their policyholder significantly improves the likelihood of a positive resolution of your claim. In your letter, you should address such things as:
- Your condition.
- It's cause.
- The progress that you have made since under chiropractic care.
- Your present status.
- Any acute episodes (frequency and cause).
- Any elements of your lifestyle that may play a role in your need for future care (hobbies, sports, childcare, stresses, or work requirements).

Although such a letter may be time consuming, it has been our experience that it is weighed very heavily by your insurance company in determining whether or not to continue to provide you with benefits.

We have already begun the process of developing our response to your insurance company. We will hold our report until we receive your letter. Please complete your letter and deliver it to our office as soon as possible so that we may include it in our reply.

Sincerely,

Michael S. Meyer, D.C.

Sample Letter: **Patient Insurance Response Letter**

The "Un-Narrative" Report

The un-narrative report that I developed several years ago has proved to be the biggest time-saver in chiropractors' offices today. As many doctors who deal with insurance or attorneys know, developing and writing the narrative reports that third parties so liberally request take time, effort, and energy. In addition, they also know that the same basic information is requested in every situation. Therefore, the following report was designed in a check-off format to allow the doctor to quickly relay the necessary details to insurance carriers and attorneys. Most of the requested information will be supplied via the examination and radiographic studies that were initially performed and are already in the patient's folder in the form of examination forms and the radiographic checklist.

Whenever a narrative report is requested (and paid for) the CA should pull the patient's file and attach all pertinent information from it. He or she will then place these materials (with the check from the requesting party) on the doctor's desk. The doctor can then review the attach copies of the appropriate forms and quickly and easily check off the appropriate information. Usually, this takes less than 15 minutes of the doctor's time to complete.

If the company requesting the narrative is adamant it wants the report in a narrative format, the doctor can simply dictate from the form and the information in the case file, using the form as a template.

Step 4-6: Effectively Handling Workers' Compensation

Just as the term "workers' compensation" implies, the injured employee in every state is entitled to various degrees of compensation whenever such an injury occurs while the employee is "on the job." Usually this compensation takes the form of payment for care of injuries sustained on the job, and for reimbursement of wages lost because of such an injury. It must be emphasized that workers' compensation laws vary greatly from state to state, and that in designing any procedure or policy in caring for an injured employee, the applicable laws in your state should be consulted. In every instance that I have witnessed, however, the workers' compensation patient must have written authori-

Patient Case Review

To: _____	Re:
_____	Patient: _____
_____	ID#: _____

SUBJECTIVE HISTORY & CHIEF COMPLAINTS	See Attached:	☐ ☐ ☐ ☐ ☐ ☐	Patient Information Form New Patient Consultation Personal Injury Questionaire Workers Compensation Questionaire Established Patient Update Form Other:_____
OBJECTIVE FINDINGS & EXAMINATION	See Attached:	☐ ☐ ☐ ☐ ☐ ☐	Subluxation Examination Form Progressive Examination & Evaluation Surface EMG Report Computerized Vertebral Compliance Report & Graph Thermographic Report Other:_____
RADIOGRAPHIC EVALUATION	See Attached:	☐ ☐ ☐	Roentgenological Report Form X-ray studies: _____ _____ Other:_____
ANALYSIS & DIAGNOSIS	ICDA CODE 1. _____ 2. _____ 3. _____ 4. _____ 5. _____		ANALYSIS _____ _____ _____ _____ _____
PLAN FOR PATIENT CARE	SHORT TERM GOALS:	☐ ☐ ☐ ☐ ☐ ☐	Reduction of altered vertebral alignment. Reduction of neuropathophysiological manifestations. Reduction of myopathophysiological manifestations. Stabilization of supportive paraspinal tissues. Improve aberrant spinal motion. Amelioration of chief presenting symptomatology.
	LONG TERM GOALS:	☐ ☐ ☐ ☐ ☐ ☐ ☐	Correction of Vertebral Subluxation Complex. Restoration of normal intersegmental integrity. Restoration of normal neurological functioning. Rehabilitation of intervertebral soft tissue components. Restorton of normal spinal kinesiological integrety. Restoration of normal physiological function. Other:_____
	APPROACH:	☐ ☐ ☐ ☐	Spinal chiropractic adjustment Trigger Point therapy Rehabilitative exercises Other:_____

Sample Form: **Patient Case Review**, front

◆ Create Financial Policies to Grow Your Practice ◆

Patient Case Review (Page 2)

PROGNOSIS	The Vertebral Subluxation Complex, with its attending subjective complaints & findings is of: ☐ a transient nature. The patient is expected to reach an asymptomatic state under conservative care in _____ to _____ weeks. ☐ an indefinate nature. The degree of change can only be speculative at this time regarding the reversability of the present complaint or injury. ☐ a permanent nature. The patient can onlu expect partial and/or temporary resolution of the presenting complaints. Acute episodes may be encountered, directly proportional to the the patient's level of physical and mental stresses.
EXTENUATING CIRCUMSTANCES	The following are exstenuating circumstances which complicate the patient's recovery or lead to periodic exacerbations of one or more components of the condition described in this report. ☐ Age ☐ Physical stressors ☐ Weight ☐ Psychological stressors ☐ General Debilitation ☐ Delay onset of appropriate care ☐ Tramaticaly induced structural weakness ☐ Deterioration of adaptive curves ☐ Other:_____ ☐ Stage of spinal degeneration ☐ Repititious physical activity
CLASSIFICATION OF CURRENT CONDITION	At the time of this report, the patient has attained: ☐ Complete recovery } Maximum level of improvement. No residuals. ☐ Incomplete recovery } Maximum level of revcovery has not been attained. Patient continues to make objective & subjective improvement. ☐ Partial recovery } Maximum level of improvement with incomplete spinal correction. Patient may experience unpredictable exacerbations of symptomatology.
CLASSIFICATION OF CURRENT CARE	☐ Crisis/Relief care } Reduction of presenting symptomatology. ☐ Corrective care } Reduction of Vertebral Subluxation Complex. ☐ Supportive care } Restoration of spinal stability ☐ Palliative care } Alleviation of exacerbations upon recurance.
PLAN FOR FUTURE CARE	☐ 30 days ☐ 60 days ☐ 90 days ☐ 120 days ☐ Sustained frequency of care: ____ x's per week. ☐ Continued reduction fo frequency of care as tolerated. ☐ Observation with dissmissal anticipated on ___/___/_____. ☐ Upon exacerbation only. (Pt to schedule as needed.) ☐ Patient dismissed. No need for further care anticipated.
SUBMITTED BY:	_____ _____ Doctor Date

Sample Form: **Patient Case Review, back**

zation from the employer *or* a telephone confirmation of authorization prior to initial consultation.

Once a new patient has been scheduled, and it has been determined that they are a possible workers' compensation case, the employer must be contacted immediately after the appointment has been made. The purpose of such a contact is to establish whether the employer has authorized the patient to receive care in this office.

Here's a possible script:

CA: "May I speak to the person in charge of workers' compensation authorization? This is Carol at Dr. Meyer's office. Your employee, Mary Jones, has just made an appointment at our office and stated that this is for an on-the-job injury. I needed to know if she has properly reported this injury, and if we will be authorized to care for her under workers' comp."

If the employer says, "Yes"—all is well. However, it is advisable to inform the employer that you are going to fax them an authorization form, and ask that it be completed and faxed back prior to the time of the patient's appointment. If the employer denies authorization, the new patient should be called immediately and informed that authorization has been denied before the employee comes into the office:

CA: "Mrs. Jones, this is Carol from Dr. Meyer's office calling. Your employer has denied authorization for us to take care of you under workers' compensation. We would still be happy to see you tomorrow though. You could utilize the benefits under your group insurance policy, if you have one, or you may wish to check with your employer and call us back."

Proper *written authorization* absolutely must be obtained from the employer prior to the patient seeing the doctor on the second visit. If a facsimile authorization has not been received from the employer, then, before the patient leaves on the first day, the patient should be given another workers' compensation authorization form and requested to return it after having it properly completed by the employer. The patient should also be informed that without this form, the doctor will not be able to see the patient at the next visit. With proper verbal em-

◆ Create Financial Policies to Grow Your Practice ◆

Authorization To Care For Injured Employee

TO: _____
_____
_____
Ph: _____

RE: Employee: _____
Date Of Injury: _____
Place: _____

This is your authorization to render care to the above named employee in accordance with, and under the conditions prescribed by the Worker's Compensation Act of the state of jurisdiction for this injury.

This care shall be only for injuries that were reported to have been sustained during the course of employment.

WORKERS COMP
NAME: _____
ADDRESS: _____
CITY: _____
STATE/ZIP: _____
PHONE: _____

EMPLOYER
NAME: _____
ADDRESS: _____
CITY: _____
STATE/ZIP: _____
PHONE: _____

Authorized By: _____ Title: _____ Date: _____

Sample Form: **Authorization to Care for Injured Employee** ployer authorization for the first visit, no payments should be collected from the patient.

Pre-Injury Status Dilemma

The biggest problem most doctors run into (and which causes problems between the doctor and the insurance adjustor) is that it is often difficult to establish when the patient is returned to a pre-injury status. Although it is often difficult for the doctor to judge, special attention during consultation to the presence of preexisting conditions and clear, up-front communication as to the responsibilities of the workers' compensation insurance carrier will help to prevent subsequent misunderstandings from occurring.

Remember, the injured employee should be cared for just like every other new patient in your office. The only difference is that you must be aware during the case report to differentiate for the patient who will be financially responsible for the different objectives of care that we will discuss in a later section.

Letter to Injured Employee

An excellent way to reinforce this distinction is to send the injured patient a "welcome to the practice" letter geared toward further explanation of the workers' compensation case. The adjacent example will help the patient understand the nature of the care in your office, and ease the inevitable transition from "work comp" to private pay or group coverage.

Dismissal Letter to Injured Employee

At some point in the future, the patient will, hopefully, reach a pre-injure status. After thoroughly reevaluating the patient and confirming that they have reached a pre-injury status and are ready to be released from workers' compensation, the doctor should explain to the patient that they are at the point where the employer's workers' compensation insurance is no longer liable for their care. At this point you should review your earlier discussion with the patient of the responsibilities of the employer and the prospects of moving into a healthcare or a wellness program of care.

If you have communicated these concepts to the patient throughout the period of condition-based care, and have educated the patient

Dear Injured Patient:

Once again, I would like to take this opportunity to welcome you to our practice. The confidence that you and your employer have placed in my staff and I is a great compliment and an immense responsibility

When a new patient enters our practice with an injury such as yours, our early attention and energies are focused on analyzing and diagnosing your injury, and then initiating a well-planned, effective program of care.

To this point, we have located the injury that appears to be the cause of your complaints. And, we are beginning to take the necessary steps to return you to a pain-free status.

Because you have suffered a work-related injury, and your employer has authorized care in our office, the insurance carrier for your employer is responsible for all costs associated with returning you to a "pre-injury" status. When we have determined that you are at the point that you were prior to the injury, you will be released from our care.

As we work together during the weeks to come, please feel free to bring to my attention any questions or problems you may have. Also, should an emergency arise after hours, please don't hesitate to call me at home when necessary. I promise that my staff and I will do all that is necessary to restore your health and to provide a warm, welcome environment that you will want to recommend to your friends and family.

Sincerely,

Michael S. Meyer, D.C.

Sample Letter: **Workers Compensation Welcome Letter**

about the true benefits of chiropractic, the patient will welcome this milestone in their healthcare. You should then send a letter reinforcing their dismissal from workers' compensation, just so there are no misunderstandings. The following is an example of the type and tone to use.

Dear Injured Patient:

As you know, we have been seeing you in our office as a result of an injury that you suffered in a work-related incident. In accordance with state law, your worker's compensation insurance carrier has been responsible for all care required returning you to a "pre-injury" status.

In reviewing your latest examination results, I am pleased to report that you have made substantial improvement, and it appears that, by all objective signs, your health has returned to the point that you were before your on-the-job injury. Therefore, I must now inform your insurance carrier that the corrective care for your work-related injuries is complete, and notify them that you have accordingly been dismissed from active care.

Speaking for myself, and my entire staff, I would like to thank you for the opportunity that you have given us to serve you. We hope that you will personally thank your employer for allowing us this opportunity.

Now that you are familiar with us, and the benefits of chiropractic health care, we hope that you will continue as one of our most valued, established patients.

Even though you have been officially dismissed from care, I want you to continue to think of me as your doctor, and I hope that you will continue to call upon us for your future healthcare needs.

Sincerely,

Michael S. Meyer, D.C.

Sample Letter: **Workers Comp Release Letter**

◆ Create Financial Policies to Grow Your Practice ◆

Key Points

- ◆ The establishment of clear and reasonable financial procedures greatly simplifies what could otherwise be a frustrating aspect of office management.
- ◆ To avoid confusion and "buck passing" there must be one person in the office who is both designated and highly trained to handle all financial arrangements with the patient.
- ◆ Financial policies describing acceptable arrangements are an absolute necessity for the CA to function effectively.
- ◆ Failure of the staff to collect from the patient or failure to enforce the agreed-upon arrangements hurts both the patient as well as the practice.
- ◆ The doctor must get a firm commitment from the patient to follow through with the recommended care. Such a commitment will make the CA's job of making arrangements and following thorough with collections straightforward and effortless.
- ◆ The patient must know they are contracting with you for their services and that you expect payment in full, on a timely basis, regardless of any settlement with a third party.
- ◆ The personal injury patient is a patient who will consume much of your time and energy in dealing with their pain, documentation, reports, depositions, and court appearances.
- ◆ By involving a patient in dealing with their insurance company, and getting them to spend the time and energy writing a letter, that individual will understand how much time and effort is involved for the doctor, as well as how unfair and uncooperative the insurance carrier may be.
- ◆ Using a report form designed in a check-off format will allow the doctor to quickly relay the necessary details to insurance carriers and attorneys.

Solution 5

Establishing Systems for a Smooth First Visit

Becoming *the* doctor in town, or more importantly, in your patient's lives, requires making a sensational first impression and then reinforcing that impression at each visit. The importance of the patient's first visit cannot be overemphasized. Strong first impressions are powerful. For this reason, the successful practice must continually work to win over the new patient and thereby set the stage for the life-changing experience of chiropractic acceptance that will follow.

This chapter will provide you with solutions to build and fill your practice with the patients you envisioned in the exercises at the beginning of this book. Because winning over your patients will set the stage for the patient's ultimate acceptance of chiropractic and chiropractor, a life of ease or a life of dis-ease, the most important phone call any person will make is to secure a first appointment in your office. Likewise, the most important phone call the CA will encounter is that of a prospective new patient. For this reason alone, it must be handled absolutely perfectly.

Your CA's ultimate success in booking the new patient is completely dependent upon whether or not they obtain the proper information from the patient and that the patient's specific questions are answered effectively. In many cases, the caller will want questions answered before he or she will commit to an appointment. Providing answers should never be seen as a disruption in the CA's work. Instead it should be impressed upon the CA that it is one of the most important functions of the job.

Step 5-1: Anticipating the New Patient's Concerns

When a new patient phones the office for an appointment, the CA has four tasks that must be completed to make that call a success. First, and most importantly, the CA must identify the caller as a prospective new patient. Quite often, when a patient who has never been in your office calls for an appointment, he or she will not identify themselves as a new patient but will merely ask for an appointment. If the caller does not identify himself or herself, the CA should immediately ask for a name. In every case, it is extremely important that the CA knows the true status of every patient for which an appointment is being requested. Absolutely nothing is worse for the doctor, the staff, and the new patient (not to mention the other patients who are in the office at the time waiting to be adjusted) for an unexpected new patient to enter the office anticipating to be seen in a timely manner.

Because such a situation results in instant stress, the CA must use the special "patient discerning technique" described below to prevent this from happening. This technique is extremely easy to use, and does not embarrass either the CA or the patient and will prevent the "unexpected new patient" problem from occurring.

Again, if a patient calls in and the CA does not absolutely and immediately recognize them as a current patient who has been in the office in the past few months, he or she must then determine if the patient is a previously established patient or a new patient:

CA: "Mrs. Jones, when was the last time you saw Dr. Meyer?"

The two most obvious answers to this question are "Last week (last month or last year)," or "I have never been in to see the doctor." At that point, the CA will then know how to appropriately book the patient.

Establishing Systems for a Smooth First Visit

Next, the CA has to effectively answer any questions the caller may have. Sometimes these questions are about the doctor, the practice, or the doctor's techniques, and can be easily answered according to circumstances. Most commonly, however, the prospective patient will ask questions that pertain to first visit procedures, costs, and payment policies. Fortunately, the prospective new patient's questions are predictable.

Understanding that such questions will be asked, adequate planning and scripting of the answers will ensure they will never be stressful to the staff members or the prospective patient. And best of all, preplanned and well designed CA scripts will increase the odds of the caller's actually scheduling the appointment. By understanding the questions that are being asked, the information the patient wants, and by having planned and practiced the answers, the CA should be able to answer these questions so effectively as to convert 90 to 99 percent of all patient inquiries into actual appointments.

The following are the questions that are most frequently asked by prospective new patients. The CA should memorize the following scripts exactly, repeating them until he or she actually owns them and feels natural saying them to a potential patient.

"How much will it cost?"

Often the staff person thinks of this caller as someone who is just a "shopper" who is looking for the office with the lowest rates in town. We have found, however, that this is not necessarily true. Quite often the prospective new patient who is asking this question is a conscientious patient who simply wants to be prepared to make payment when he or she comes into the office, and should be treated with respect and patience.

Unfortunately, this is one of the most difficult questions for the CA to answer. The caller wants a specific dollar amount to be quoted, but until the patient is seen by the doctor, no one knows what clinical procedures or x-rays will need to be performed in the proper management of the case. Of course, the CA will not know the precise amount and should not attempt to form an opinion as to what the doctor might recommend. Therefore, the best answer in this situation is to simply be up front and explain this to the patient.

It is also helpful to design a policy for the prospective new patient where the initial costs are lowered sufficiently to allow the patient to come into the office with little or no financial risk. By establishing a lower initial consultation fee, the patient may be brought into the office, meet and discuss their concern with the doctor, and then be advised of the total anticipated cost of the initial chiropractic work-up that is indicated in their case.

Here's a possible response:

CA: "There is a $25 (or no) charge for the initial consultation. After talking to you, the doctor will have an idea as to what you might need and can then more accurately give you an idea of the procedures and tests that are indicated at that time, as well as what the initial costs of those procedures might be. We have an opening for a new patient tomorrow morning at 10:00. Would you like to make an appointment with the doctor?"

"But can't you give me some idea how much it would be?"

Usually the caller will understand and the above reply is sufficient to appoint a high percentage of these callers. Some people, however, are looking for a specific stated price for their initial visit and will continue to press for a specific answer. This is the persistent patient who really wants a dollar amount to be quoted. Since neither the doctor nor the CA will actually know the answer, the same answer as above should be given, just a little more specific and with a little different tone. It may even be appropriate, at this point, for the CA to give an upper limit fee. If such an amount is stated, great care should be made to explain that this fee is "high-end" and that the patient will possibly (probably) be charged less. (Remember…be honest, never "bait and switch.")

Here's another possible response:

CA: "There is no set fee for the initial visit. It depends on your case and what procedures might be appropriate for you. The doctor can tell you after (he or she) has had a chance to talk with you. However, I can tell you that it will not be more than $ (insert number). It is quite often less.

"Would you like to come in and just talk to the doctor? There is no charge for the initial consultation. Then, if the doctor feels that chiropractic can help you, (he or she) can then give you an idea as to the costs. If (he or she) believes that chiropractic cannot help you, (he or she) will tell you that also, and help you find someone who can."

"Will my insurance cover my care in your office?"

Here, the patient is concerned as to the amount of actual costs to them should they come into your office. A qualified blanket statement that "most" insurances do is usually reassuring to the patient. If, however, the CA is knowledgeable about the various coverages in your community he or she may further assist the patient with their knowledge about that coverage.

> *CA:* "In most cases it does. However, that depends on your policy and coverage. What insurance company do you have? Is that a group policy? Is it with your employer? Where do you work?"

"Do I have to pay when I come in?"

This question is often a tipoff that the patient does not want to make payment or to assume financial responsibility for his or her own care. A specific, straightforward answer here is appropriate:

> *CA:* "Yes, but we can make financial arrangements if necessary."

This reply should inform the patient that they are expected to assume responsibility for their care, but that at the same time, you and your practice exist to serve your patients and your community. It should also inform them that if the patient is conscientious about paying for their services, arrangements will be made for them to receive needed care.

"Do I have to be x-rayed?"

Be careful answering this questing. Many times when a patient asks this question the CA actually has no idea as to the reason behind it. The CA does not know if the patient is looking for a doctor who takes x-rays, or one who does not. The following answer will cover both callers. It will reassure the first yet while appearing reasonable to the second.

> *CA:* "No, not necessarily. But if you do need x-rays, the doctor will certainly recommend them."

"I was in a car accident. Can you just bill my insurance company?"

The answer to this question depends entirely on your decision as to the type of practice you wish to develop and what policies you will design to deal with these types of patients. If you wish to develop a personal injury practice, your answer will be "yes." If you understand that this type of patient needs chiropractic care, yet it is not your policy to deal with third parties in these types of cases, the following answer will reinforce your practice's policy yet leave the door open for the patient to receive needed care.

> **CA:** "I'm sorry, our policy is to bill the patient or the patient's group insurance, and then let the patient deal with the liable insurance company directly. We will be happy to assist you with billings and reports for your (auto) insurance company though."

Once all questions are answered, the CA must proceed to properly schedule the appointment at the appropriate time as it relates to the block-booking mandates of the office and the doctor's schedule. First, however, the CA should ask the caller for permission to give the caller an appointment.

> **CA:** "Would you like an appointment to see the doctor?"

Such a question and a resulting affirmative reply will indicate to the CA the patient's questions have been answered, and at the same time, it prevents the patient from feeling "railroaded" or pressured into making an appointment. This simple question will make a big difference in practices that have a large number of "no-show" new patient appointments.

Booking the New Patient

Once all of the patient's questions are answered, and the caller has indicated a desire to make an appointment, the CA should begin collecting the appropriate information on the patient. Experience has shown that the more information you can gather on a prospective patient, the better the odds that they will actually show up for their appointment. Therefore, the CA should ask the patient for all of the information required to complete the new patient information slip. With this infor-

♦ Establishing Systems for a Smooth First Visit ♦

mation, also, the patient's file and paperwork can be prepared before the new patient arrives—speeding up the first visit process.

CA: "Mrs. Jones, if you have a minute, I would like to get some information from you so I can get your file prepared for tomorrow."

The CA should then proceed to fill out the form, especially noting the proper spelling and pronunciation of the last name, and who referred the new patient. Not only does this slip enable the CA to collect all of the information necessary to prepare for in advance and then process the new patient. In addition, should a new patient ever fail to

---

New Patient Information

Date: _____ Time of Call: _____
Name: _____
Address: _____
           Street   City   St.   Zip
Appointment For: o Self   o Family   oOther: _____
Home Phone: _____
Work Phone: _____

Appointment Made: ☐ Mon.   ☐ Tues.   ☐ Wed.
                    ☐ Thur.   ☐ Fri.   ☐ Sat.
Time: _____   ☐ AM   ☐ PM

Referred By: _____
Family Member Patient: _____
Employer: _____
☐ Auto Accident (Attorney: _____)
☐ Work Related Injury (Reported to: _____)
☐ Group Insurance (Bring Insurance Card)
☐ Medicare
☐ Directions Given
☐ Special Questions: _____
_____

Form—16   Michael S. Meyer, D.C. 2003

Sample Form: **New Patient Information Slip**

keep an appointment (and especially if failed new patient appointments become frequent), it gives you the ability to determine which CA booked the appointment. You can further investigate if there were any procedural or personality problems that may have caused the patient to make the appointment and then not show up.

After answering the caller's questions and completing the new patient information slip, the CA should invite the caller to make an appointment. The booking of the new patient should be performed utilizing the same block-booking scheduling procedure as with any other patient, procedurally "forcing" the caller into the designated times for a new patient.

> *CA:* "Mrs. Jones. we can see you either tomorrow or Friday. Which do you prefer? Morning or afternoon? Earlier in the morning or later?"

Before ending the telephone call, the CA should give the patient directions to the office:

> *CA:* "Mrs. Jones, our office is located at (give address and directions). Can you find us?"

It also helps to give the patient an idea of how much time it will take for the first visit. Doing so allows the patient to plan for and schedule sufficient time in their schedule, thus preventing the patient from becoming stressed and worrying about other time commitments during the initial visit.

> *CA:* "You should plan on spending between 30 and 45 minutes for the first visit, so the doctor can be as thorough as possible. Do you have any other questions?"
>
> *Note:* Unless your desired type of practice resembles a hospital emergency room, or a walk-in clinic, drop-in or walk-in new patients should *never* be taken at the time they happen to come into the office. Doing so will ultimately cause the patient to believe the practice is not that busy (successful), or that your time is not to be respected. It has been demonstrated (more than once) that a walk-in new patient who is seen immediately will expect to receive care on the first visit, expect immediate relief, and whether relief is effected or not, will never become the lifelong, perfect patient that you desire.

These individuals usually represent the type of patient who is looking for a quick fix and is not committed to either correction or wellness.

Instead, if a prospective patient simply drops in without an appointment, the staff should be trained to present the patient with an option of two later times in the day or the next day to return for an appointment. If the prospective patient agrees to a future time, the CA should complete the new patient information slip, and give the new patient the initial patient information form, the family health history form, and even the financial options form to be taken with them, completed, and returned at the appointed time. Having the appropriate induction forms completed when the patient returns, will streamline the initial visit, but more importantly, gathering the information requested on the new patient information slip will help ensure the patient won't go to the next office down the road and make an appointment there.

The CA's "wowing" the prospective new patient caller is just as dependent on the CA's attitude, knowledge, and personality on the telephone as it is the actual answers given. When staffing the office, the doctor should be alert to the telephone voice, attitude, and personality of the person placed in this position. Remember, the attitude that the new patient will bring into the relationship on the first visit is in many ways dependent on how the initial call is handled.

Step 5-2: Shaping the New Patient's First Impression

When patients enter the office for the first time, they are generally concerned and nervous about the pending encounter with a new doctor. Along with their concern, they are bringing with them their worries over the prospects of losing their health. They may even be troubled over the prospect of losing their ability to work and fulfill their responsibilities in life. Moreover, they usually come in with legitimate financial concerns—especially if they have recently been unable to work. Add all of these concerns to the apprehension of seeing a strange new doctor for the first time, and you can appreciate the level of stress that a new patient may bring with them into your office on the first visit.

More than likely, they hold such apprehensions based on whatever past experiences they may have had with other doctors. Such experiences were, in all probability, not favorable. They may not have been treated with due respect. The doctor may have been aloof, unconcerned.

Maybe the doctor's level of professional skill was not up to par. In all likelihood the staff was cold, distant, improperly trained, and treated them as interruptions. Or worse, they might have had to wait a "long" time to see the doctor.

These, and many more concerns, are in the minds of most new patients as they enter your office. It has been said that "a bad first impression is hard to overcome" but the truth is that most patients have a poor image and a bad first impression of all doctors' offices. Many may carry adversarial attitudes when they first enter your office.

Because of this, from the initial phone call to the time they leave on the first visit, every procedure, every point of patient contact must be designed to overcome a bad first impression or an adversarial attitude whether your office has caused it or not.

Our first goal with a new patient is always to surprise and to disarm the patient with warmth, understanding, and efficiency the minute they enter the office. Doing so, is easy, and the results can be dramatic. How? Just treat the new patient as you would like to be treated. This attitude must be a team effort. Every person in the office who has even the slightest contact with the patient is an important member of your new patient team. Every procedure that will be described is designed to "wow" the patient, to make them feel recognized, approved of, and appreciated.

For the ultimate success of your practice, and eventually the patient's success in achieving good health under your care, that first impression had better be a good one. Changing the patient's impression of your practice as merely a "doctor's office" will set the stage for many wonderful results. It is the first step in practice building and practice growth, but, most importantly, it may determine whether or not patients will accept your recommendations and allow themselves to experience the greatest opportunity of their lives to regain and maintain their health and ultimately the health of their entire family. Therefore, the very first impression of your office will color each and every action and reaction the patient will have from that point and ultimately determine the success of every activity and interaction that will follow.

The new patient's initial entrance into the office is the most crucial point of contact in the office/patient relationship. Every patient entering your office for the first time will quickly analyze the office and the

Establishing Systems for a Smooth First Visit

staff's appearance, their friendliness, thoroughness, other patients in the office. In fact, researchers tell us that the patient's first impression of your office and staff will usually be formed in the first three to five minutes. It is during these first minutes that the patient decides either consciously or subconsciously how they are going to react to and accept you.

If you and your staff do not present yourselves in a positive, professional manner to the new patient, or if you do not adhere to the procedures necessary to win the patient's confidence, it will directly affect the quality and quantity of the practice. It also may be directly responsible for that patient not following through with needed care and thus being fated to a life of pain and sickness because of the failure to get the necessary chiropractic care.

New Patient Hospitality

When expecting a new patient, the staff must be aware and watchful for the person when they enter the office. When the new patient approaches the front desk for the first time, it is important that any staff members present acknowledge the arrival immediately, call the person by name, and show warmth, respect, and professionalism. Immediate eye contact and a reassuring smile are the CA's greatest assets in making the new patient feel welcome.

> **CA:** "Hello, Mrs. Jones, welcome to our office. My name is Carol. I spoke with you yesterday. I am happy to meet you in person (CA should stand up and shake hands with patient). If you would please sign in and then have a seat, I will get your file and we will be ready for you."

At this point, the CA should let the patient sit in the reception room for one to two minutes to give the person the chance to acclimate to the office. The CA should then go out and sit down next to the patient with a clipboard and the proper forms to be completed. (patient information form, financial options form, and informed consent form) The CA should then explain what each form is for and show the patient where to sign them. When the paperwork is done, the patient should be taken back to the consultation area where the doctor will perform the clinical portion of the visit.

Step 5-3: Assembling the Initial New Patient Information

After welcoming the new patient into the office and into the practice, it is necessary to begin the process of gathering all the information that will be needed for you to care for the patient and to manage their case properly. At the same time, it is important to begin to prepare the patient to understand the various office policies that have been established.

Personal and Historical Information

The new patient information form is designed for efficiency and thoroughness in gathering the proper information on the new patient. This form will compile all of the personal information necessary to establish a patient file, as well as give the doctor and staff the basic information needed to understand this patient's case. It should be the first item the new patient is asked to complete upon entering the office.

The first section of this form includes all pertinent personal and health information needed to give the doctor an accurate overall picture of the patient before actually entering the room for the initial consultation. The form is complete in its gathering of appropriate information, yet simple enough that the new patient can complete it in less than 15 minutes.

The current health concern section is designed to give the doctor an immediate overview of the presenting complaint. You must remember, however, that the patient is only asked about the primary entrance complaint on this form. It is your duty to follow up with an in-depth consultation digging for other complaints as well as previous injuries and chronicity.

The second side of the patient information form delves into any other health issues with which the patient may be dealing. It also provides a systematic check of the patient's total health picture.

Finally, there is an important section where the patient is asked to mark the actual areas of their complaints. It is vitally important that this section is completed. A schematic depiction of the complaint is always more accurate than the patient's verbal description, which is subject to interpretation by the doctor.

◆ Establishing Systems for a Smooth First Visit ◆

New Patient Information
(Please Complete As Thoroughly As Possible)

Personal Information

Name:_____ Spouse:_____

Address:_____ City_____ State:____ Zip:_____

Home Phone:_____ Date of Birth:_____ SS#:_____ - ____ - _____

Age:_____ Sex: ☐ M ☐ F Marital Status: ☐ M ☐ S ☐ W ☐ D

Employer:_____ Work Phone:_____

Type of Work Performed:_____

In Case Of Emergency Notify:_____ Phone #:_____

Who Is Your Family Physician?_____

Who Should We Thank For Telling You About Our Office?_____

Current Health Concern

Primary Reason For Today's Visit?_____

Check The Severity Of Your Complaint: (Mild) ☐ ☐ ☐ ☐ ☐ ☐ ☐ ☐ ☐ (Severe)

When Did This Begin?_____ Experienced Previously? ☐ Yes ☐ Never

Is This Condition: ☐ Job Related ☐ Auto Accident ☐ Fall or Injury ☐ Other:_____

Other Doctors Seen For This Problem? _____

Other Doctor's Opinions or Diagnosis? _____

Other Or Secondary Health Concerns:_____

Drugs Or Medications Now Taking: ☐ Pain Killers / Muscle Relaxants   ☐ Tranquilizers
                                  ☐ Blood Pressure Medicine   ☐ Antibiotics
                                  ☐ Other:_____

Past Health History

Previous Surgeries: ☐ Eyes / Ears / Nose / Throat   ☐ Head / Neck   ☐ Back / Spine
                    ☐ Chest / Heart / Lungs   ☐ Abdominal   ☐ Other:_____

Previous Fractures Or Broken Bones: ☐ Yes ☐ No Describe:_____

Previous Falls Or Accidents: ☐ Yes ☐ No Describe:_____

Previoius Hospitalization: ☐ Yes ☐ No Describe:_____

Previous Chiropractic Care: ☐ Yes ☐ No Describe:_____

Similar Problem In Family?   ☐ Yes ☐ No Describe:_____

Similar Problems With Co-workers?   ☐ Yes ☐ No Describe:_____

Do You Workout Or Exercise?   ☐ Yes ☐ No Describe:_____

Sample Form: **New Patient Information (front)**

◆ 7 Solutions for Building Your Proactive Chiropractic Practice ◆

Patient Information (Side 2)

Check Any Of The Following That Applies To You

Health Issues:

- ☐ Polio
- ☐ Cancer
- ☐ Diabetes
- ☐ High Stress
- ☐ Under Weight
- ☐ Arthritis
- ☐ AIDS or ARC
- ☐ Frequent Illnesses
- ☐ Poor Diet
- ☐ Other:_____
- ☐ Diabetes
- ☐ Heart
- ☐ Allergies
- ☐ Epilepsy
- ☐ Sleeplessness
- ☐ Chronic Fatigue
- ☐ Genetic Disorders
- ☐ Over Weight

Intake Or Use:

- ☐ Alcohol
- ☐ Sleeping Pills
- ☐ Tobacco
- ☐ Other:_____
- ☐ Pain Relievers
- ☐ Caffiene

Check Any Problems That You May Have Had Within The Past Six Months

Muscles—Skeleton

- ☐ Low Back Pain
- ☐ Middle Back
- ☐ Neck
- ☐ Shoulders / Arms
- ☐ Joint Pain / Stiffness
- ☐ Hips / Legs

Circulation—Breathing

- ☐ Chest
- ☐ Lungs / Breathing
- ☐ Blood Pressure
- ☐ Heart Rate
- ☐ Chest Pain
- ☐ Sinus Pain

Eye—Ear—Nose—Throat

- ☐ Eyes / Vision
- ☐ Dental / TMJ
- ☐ Throat / Voice
- ☐ Ears / Hearing
- ☐ Sinus

Nerve System

- ☐ Headaches
- ☐ Nervousness
- ☐ Numbness / Tingling
- ☐ Muscle Weakness
- ☐ Dizziness
- ☐ Forgetfulness
- ☐ Depression
- ☐ Fainting
- ☐ Seizures
- ☐ Cold Hands / Feet
- ☐ Stress Reactions
- ☐ Shaking / Tremors

Digestion—Elimination

- ☐ Poor Appetite
- ☐ Excessive Thirst
- ☐ Nausea
- ☐ Diarrhea
- ☐ Constipation
- ☐ Hemorrhoids
- ☐ Weight Loss / Gain
- ☐ Heartburn
- ☐ Change In Stools

Urinary—Genitals

- ☐ Pain With Urination
- ☐ Infrequent Urination
- ☐ Frequent Urination
- ☐ Weak Stream
- ☐ Bladder Control
- ☐ Genitals

Female Only

- ☐ Menstrual
- ☐ Low Back W/ Per.
- ☐ Pain With Urination
- ☐ Breast

Please Mark Area Of Concern

Are You Pregnant? ☐ Yes ☐ No

(X) Pain
(O) Spasm
(-) Numb

I understand that my care in this office may involve the making of judgements that are based upon the facts known by the doctor. Therfore, the above information is true and complete to the best of my knowledge. I also understand that the practice of any healing art is not an exact science and that no guarantee of results will be made by the doctor nor relied upon by me. I furhter understand that the doctor's professional expertise lies in detecting and correcting the structural and mechanical abberations of the spine - the Vertebral Subluxation Complex. I agree that I will not hold the doctor responsible for the diagnosis or treatment of any medical condition indicated above.

Patient's Signature:

Sample Form: **New Patient Information (back)**

◆ Establishing Systems for a Smooth First Visit ◆

Patient Financial Options

Our practice provides two options for the handling of our patient's financial accounts. Please review the following choices and check the type of arrangement that best depicts the way you would like us to handle your account.

Thank-you!

☐ Approved Insurance Option

The following policy applies to those patients with approved health insurance coverage. (We do not accept assignment on personal injury nor secondary insurance benefits.)

1. We will accept assignment on the estimated amount of insurance benefits available through the patient's primary insurance carrier.

2. Our office will estimate the total cost of care, and pro-rate the patients portion into a weekly payments

3. Only patients undergoing active initial intensive care will be eligible to assign their insurance benefits to this office.

4. If the patient discontinues care prior to being released by doctor, all outstanding balances will immediately become due and payable.

☐ Non-Insured / Cash Option

The following policy applies to those patients who do not have health insurance benefits or to those who prefer to pay for their services and handle their own insurance processing.

1. Our office does not bill patients for their care. Payment is expected at time of service.

2. We accept cash, check, MasterCard, and VISA as payment for services rendered.

3. We will not deny care to anyone based on their inability to pay for our services.

4. If necessary, we will make arrangements with patients who may be experiencing financial difficulties and who request that such arrangements be made.

5. We will provide forms, information, and the guidance to enable patients to process their own insurance claims if they so desire.

Patient or Guardian:_____ Date:_____

Sample Form: **Patient Financial Options**

The Patient Payment Options Form

The next component of proper patient induction is to identify how the patient expects to handle their financial obligations. Placing the simple and straightforward patient payment options form on the clipboard for the patient to complete serves two important functions. First, it informs the CA as to how to properly handle the patient's finances without having to ask. This saves the CA from having to broach the discussion of fees until after the patient has had a chance to be "wowed" by the doctor and staff. Concurrently, knowing how to proceed with the new patient on a financial level is important in how the CA will prepare the paperwork and make collections for the first visit.

Also, this form effectively gives the patient early information on practice financial policies. It notifies the patient that there are two acceptable forms of managing finances. At the same time, it gives the patient an option as to which approach best suits their needs. Allowing patients to select either of the options removes the heavy-handed approach so often associated with the presentation of set policies yet establishes the policies firmly in their consciousness. Having the prospective patient select either of these options immediately brings the patient into agreement with the stated office policies regarding payment before ever confronting a staff person.

The Informed Consent Form

The third form to be placed on the clipboard for the new patient to complete is the Doctor-Patient Relationship and Informed Consent form. In most cases, the patient will simply sign this form with no further questions being asked. Nevertheless, even with the form read and signed, the doctor must explain all of the parameters of the patient's case and obtain consent prior to accepting the case. If the patient has any question pertaining to the form or hesitates in signing it, the CA should graciously acknowledge that reluctance and let the doctor handle the issue of "informed consent" with the patient, after the consultation and prior to the examination.

A well-designed informed consent form helps start the doctor-patient relationship out on the right foot. It is more than simply a statement spelling out the possible adverse side effects of any given procedure, as most people believe. It acknowledges and describes the difference be-

◆ Establishing Systems for a Smooth First Visit ◆

Informed Consent
And The Doctor-Patient Relationship

Chiropractic Care	It is the premise of Chiropractic that the human body possesses the inherent potential to maintain itself in a natural state of homeostasis. A state of normal homeostasis allows the body to establish normal function, express appropriate adaptation, and employ its recuperative, health sustaining powers. The relationship between the spine and the nervous system may affect the conduction of the nerve impulses over the nervous system affecting that inherent potential. Therefore, chiropractic care focuses primarily on the chiropractic adjustment for the purpose of establishing proper spinal alignment thus allowing normal nerve conduction throughout the body. The success of chiropractic care often depends on the environment, underlying causes and the physical and spinal conditions of each individual patient.
Chiropractic Analysis	The doctor will conduct a clinical analysis for the express purpose of determining the presence of the vertebral subluxation and the effects of the vertebral subluxation complex. If such is not detected, the patient will be informed and an attempt to refer the patient to an appropriate health care provider will be made.
Clinical Results	The purpose of chiropractic care is to promote health though the correction of the vertebral subluxation complex. Since there are so many variables, it is difficult to predict the time schedule, degree of response, or the efficacy of the chiropractic adjustment for any given patient. However, the doctor may make recommendations for clinical management based upon known circumstances and clinical experience. Due to the complexities of nature, and the many variables (both known and unknown) that can affect a patient's response, no doctor can promise specific results. The Doctor of Chiropractic is licensed to provide a specialized unique, non-duplicating heath service. The Chiropractor is licensed in a special area of practice and is available to work with other providers in your health care regimen.
Medical Diagnosis	Although Doctors of Chiropractic are experts in the analysis of the structural alignment of the human spine and its effects on the nervous system, they are not internal medical or surgical specialists. Therefore, every patient should be mindful of their own symptoms and should secure other opinions should they have any concerns as to the nature of any other symptoms or their total health picture. Your Doctor of Chiropractic may express an opinion as to whether or not further consultation is necessary, but the patient is responsible for the final decision and any subsequent action.
Informed Consent For Chiropractic Care	Where vertebral subluxations are detected, the chiropractic adjustment is usually beneficial and seldom causes any adverse reactions. In rare cases, undetected physical defects, deformities, or pathologies may render the patient susceptible to such injuries as vascular accidents, fractures and disc injury. The doctor, of course, will not perform any procedures if there is an awareness that such care may be contra-indicated. Again, it is the responsibility of the patient to make it known or to learn through other health care providers whether they are suffering from: pathological conditions (latent or otherwise), illnesses, injuries, or deformities which otherwise not come to the attention of this doctor. By signing below, the patient affirms that they have been open and truthful in disclosing their health history, and gives the doctor permission and authority to examine and care for them in accordance with recognized standards and acceptable chiropractic analytical and corrective procedures.
Patient Consent	Please discuss any questions or problems with the doctor before signing this statement of understanding and consent for care. I have read and understand the foregoing. I hereby request and authorize the doctor to render chiropractic care to me: _____ _____ Signature of Patient, Parent, or Guardian Date

Sample Form: **Informed Consent**

tween the healthcare specialties of chiropractic, osteopathy, and allopathic medicine. It is also helps the patient understand the premises and principals of chiropractic and what to expect from chiropractic care. When presenting the form to the patient to sign, the CA should encourage the patient to read it in its entirety.

The informed consent should also address the type of clinical analysis that will be performed and that this analysis will determine whether the patient's presenting complaint is the result of a vertebral subluxation...which would then qualify the patient as an excellent prospect for chiropractic care.

Some careful discussion of the results expected may be addressed as well. The document should address the fact that many variables exist in case management and that it is difficult to predict the time schedule or the effectiveness of the chiropractic adjustment on any given patient. The informed consent should also mention that results are sometimes less than expected.

A clause describing the specialization of the doctor in the analysis of the structural alignment of the human spine and its effects on the nerve system may be included. The form also should state that the doctor is not an internal medical specialist, and that every patient should be mindful of their own symptoms and should secure other opinions if they have any special concerns as to the nonchiropractic aspects of their condition.

The patient should then be asked to sign this document, giving the doctor permission and authority to care for him or her in accordance with recognized and acceptable chiropractic analytical and corrective procedures. Finally, the actual informed consent portion of the document should state that, in rare cases, undetected physical defects, deformities, or pathologies may render the patient susceptible to injury. The patient should be counseled that the doctor, of course, will not give an adjustment if he or she is aware that such care might be contraindicated.

♦ Establishing Systems for a Smooth First Visit ♦

Step 5-4: Establishing a Procedure to Verify the Patient's Insurance Coverage

Although many patients do have group or personal health insurance coverage, today's policies are so varied in their benefits that specific coverage should never be taken for granted. For this reason, it is essential that the CA contact the insurance carrier prior to the initiation of care to determine and verify policy coverage, amounts, and limitations.

After the new patient completes the new patient information form, the CA should immediately note if the cash option or insurance option is checked on the financial options form. If "insurance" was checked, the CA should immediately ask the patient for an insurance card before taking the patient to the examination room.

>**CA:** "Mrs. Jones, I see you have marked the 'insurance option' on your form. Do you have your insurance card with you?"

From the card, the CA can then obtain the insured's name, policy numbers, plus the address and phone number of the insurance company. Ideally, a photocopy of the card should be taken on the back of the Insurance Verification Worksheet at this time. (Minimally, all information on the card should be written down.)

>*Note:* Any patient who cannot produce an insurance card will be considered a cash patient until one is produced and coverage is verified.

Once the patient has been taken back for the initial consultation and examination with the doctor, the CA should call the insurance company to verify the limits of coverage. The insurance company's telephone number can usually be found on the patient's insurance card. The following dialog will help ensure that the CA gathers all of the necessary information to successfully file for and receive insurance benefits:

>**CA:** "I would like to verify coverage on one of your policy holders..."
>
>(Wait for a response.)
>
>"I am sorry; I did not catch your name...?"
>
>"May I have your extension number, please?"
>
>(Verify coverage.)

"Is there coverage for chiropractic care in this plan?

"Are there any policy limits or restrictions?

"Could you tell me what the deductible and coinsurance are on this policy?

"Has the deductible been met for this year?

"What is the coverage after deductible has been met?"

The CA may then continue to complete the Insurance Verification Worksheet. It is important to remember that the verification of insurance information is a service provided by the carrier and it is never to be considered adversarial in nature. The caller must always be friendly and professional in their demeanor. The chances are high that he or she will be requesting information for this same person at some future date.

Step 5-5: Developing a Strong Doctor-Patient Relationship

Besides gathering the important clinical information necessary to properly care for the new patient, developing a strong doctor-patient relationship on the initial visit is critical. If the patient is to accept the doctor on a personal level plus the doctor's recommendations for care, the seeds of a strong relationship must be planted early. Luckily, the thorough and professional gathering of that same clinical information greatly augments the development of the relationship. These activities, when enhanced by a doctor whose personality and demeanor are warm, compassionate, and truly concerned, will set the proper environment for acceptance, compliance, and healing to occur.

Introducing the Concept of "Transition Statements"

When inducting a new patient into the practice, there are five specific points of interaction and procedural steps that must be carried out to properly assess and qualify the patient during the initial visit. These five steps include:

1. The initial consultation
2. The new patient examination
3. The new patient x-rays
4. The first visit release
5. The second visit post-adjustment release

Each of these specific steps must be introduced to the patient and the intrinsic value of each procedure thoroughly explained. The benefit of properly describing each procedure, and its necessity, constitutes the first steps toward securing patient compliance and in laying the foundation for effective patient education. In addition, taking the time for such descriptions will ultimately establish an attitude of trust and acceptance on the part of the patient. Giving the patient such information and repeatedly gaining the patient's permission to proceed will likely form the basis for a rewarding doctor-patient partnership in the early days of care, as well as create the foundation for a great relationship for years to come.

Therefore, as you implement the following new patient induction strategies, I urge you to develop specific, well-designed, and effortlessly presented statements that will "transition" the patient though every step of their first visit. The statements that will be used to bring the patient through these points of transition are called "transition statements." As we discuss each step of the new patient processing in this chapter we will also discuss all five of the transition statements individually.

At each of the five steps we will give suggestions for effective transition statements. I suggest that you review them carefully and use them if they feel comfortable to you. You should also feel free to design your own statements that are consistent with your practice, your procedures, and your personality. In the end, the goal is to make certain that your communication is educating the patient, while gaining their permission and making them an active participant as you proceed through each step of their induction into your practice.

The Initial Consultation and Relationship Building

The initial consultation is truly the launching of the doctor-patient relationship. It is here that the new patient solidifies their first impressions of the doctor, the office, and the appropriateness and rationale of the clinical procedures. And, most importantly, by the end of the consultation they should have a strong impression of the doctor's competence.

Although first impressions may be the most lasting, with a little planning they can also be the most controllable. There is no question that how you handle this encounter will set the stage for every other undertaking between you and the patient throughout the entire relationship.

During the initial visit, the doctor must always keep in mind that while assessing the patient on a physical plane, the patient is evaluating the doctor on an emotional and possibly irrational level. Every aspect of the doctor and the practice is being assimilated, filtered, and evaluated by every new patient, based upon their perceptions of how they compare to other doctors and offices they have experienced.

The patient may wonder: "Is this doctor a nice person?" "Will this doctor care about me?" "Will this doctor take the time to get to know me and understand my problem?" "Will this doctor ask the right questions or just blow me off?"

These questions make up the cross currents of thoughts that run through the patient's mind before and during the consultation. For better or worse, one way or another, by the end of the consultation, those questions will have been answered. How those questions are answered will set the stage for the degree to which the patient will accept the doctor and ultimately embrace and follow his or her recommendations.

Yes, both you and the patient ask and answer many questions about each other during the first visit. Unfortunately, the patient's questions must be anticipated because they are often unspoken. While the doctor is developing the facts of the patient's health concerns, the patient is simultaneously drawing important conclusions about the doctor. Subconsciously patients are forming opinions about the doctor's degree of caring and competence; whether or not they will pay for their care; if they will remain under care; what they will tell others about their new doctor and the office.

Most of these patient issues will all be decided during the consultation. Therefore, it can be argued that success in practice is ultimately determined by the first impressions the patient develops during the first 10 to 15 minutes of their relationship with the doctor and staff.

Establishing Systems for a Smooth First Visit

Therefore, the main objective during the first visit must be for the doctor to present him- or herself as a competent and caring doctor and clinician. When the first visit is complete, it is the consultation and examination that will have the patient leaving the office thinking: "Wow. They know my problems…they understand me…and they care about me…."

Most of us who have been in practice for a while understand that new patients have already tried everything else before making their first appointment in a chiropractic office. They have tolerated pain for weeks, maybe months, before seeking our help. They have waited to see if the pain will go away. They have taken all of the over-the-counter drugs they have seen advertised on television. They probably have already been to their "regular" doctor. Although the patients may be scared and skeptical, they are also in pain and ill-health. Because of this, they are at the point where they are willing to risk putting their health and their future into a stranger's hands by consulting a new or at least different kind doctor.

The most critical thought for you to keep in mind is that (except in rare occurrences) it is *always* the *symptom* that initially brings the patient to your office. Whatever the problem is, the doctor must always remember that it is significant and threatening to the patient who seeks your care. After days, weeks, or months of suffering, the patient has finally come to the conclusion that his or her lifestyle, family life, and ability to earn a living are at risk—threatened by the pain and symptoms for which no relief has been provided or explanation afforded. This is why, above all else, the patient must know that you fully understand and empathize with them and their complaint. If you are to be successful with this patient, never act like the complaint is unimportant, inconsequential, or routine.

During the consultation, you have a precious opportunity to show the patient you are competent and that you care. Both are important prerequisites in successful patient management. In short, it is the consultation that either makes or breaks the doctor-patient relationship. No matter how much you care, if you do not do a thorough consultation, do not ask pertinent questions, and do not show signs of utmost concern, the patient will (either consciously or unconsciously) feel that you are uncaring and/or incompetent, and that you do not understand their problems. They will resent you, and ultimately find another doctor who does show the concern and compassion they need and demand by asking the right questions.

First Step in Successful Risk Management

In today's litigious environment, it is not enough to have a perfunctory idea of the patient's primary and secondary complaints and then initiate care. For your personal and professional sake, you need to know every detail of the patient's presenting complaints. Nothing should be omitted or overlooked. Without a good consultation, you cannot be a good doctor. If you are not perceived as a good doctor, you will not care for the large number of people who need your services, nor will you be as successful as you would have been otherwise.

Transition Statement One: Pre-Consultation

Before delving into the new patient consultation you must explain to the patient how important it is for you to know everything there is to know about his or her current health and health history. Transitioning from meeting the patient to getting down to business is extremely important. In fact, it sets the tone for the rest of your relationship with that patient. It shows that as a doctor (and a human being) you are caring, thorough, and, most of all, honest.

When you first meet the new patient, it is important that you introduce yourself and make the patient feel welcome and at ease. A loving/caring demeanor with a firm, two-handed handshake, good eye contact, and a sincere smile are usually the only tools necessary. Be yourself, be relaxed, and be sincere. Don't overdo it or the patient will see you as a fake.

Study this script and memorize it:

Doctor: "Hello, Mrs. Jones. Welcome to our practice, I am Dr. Meyer. I am happy to meet you. I see by your entry form that you are having some (name symptoms) problems."

(Listen intently to the patient's initial response.) "Before we begin, let me give you an idea of what to expect today. We see many patients with (name symptoms). Unfortunately, the actual causes of these symptoms are as varied as the patients themselves.

"Therefore, our main goal today is to find out what is causing your problems. To do so, we need to perform a thorough health history and a chiropractic examination. If indicated, we may need to get some x-rays.

"If I can find the actual cause of your (name symptoms), then I will have a good idea if chiropractic can help you or not. If it appears that yours is a chiropractic case I will do everything possible to resolve your concerns.

"However, if yours is not a chiropractic case, I will be the first person to tell you that and I will help you find someone who can help you. Is that fair enough?"

(Wait for patient to nod or give their consent.)

"First, let's make sure that I understand the problems you are experiencing."

(Proceed with consultation by completing the Patient Consultation Worksheet.)

Step 5-6: Being an Interested, Active Listener—the Consultation

The patient's initial consultation will be performed using the Patient Consultation Worksheet. This important tool will give you the means to keep the consultation on track and to efficiently obtain all the information that will give you a clear picture of this patient's health concerns. Great effort should be made to complete this form in as much detail as possible. Being interested, thorough, and asking the right questions is not only good doctoring, it lets the patient know you are concerned and working hard to gather all the information possible, to make informed decisions and render fact-based recommendations.

Following are the nine basic components of a thorough consultation. Omit any one of them, and your consultation is incomplete. Discuss each section with the patient and you will have a complete picture of the patient and the problem that has led them to seek you out.

1. Symptoms or Complaints. First, you must begin where the patient expects you to begin. Therefore, you need an accurate description of the patient's actual symptoms. How does the patient describe the com-

7 Solutions for Building Your Proactive Chiropractic Practice

New Patient Consultation
(Worksheet)

Patient:_____ Date:_____

Symptoms & Complaints

Primary Complaint:_____ Degree: ☐ Mild ☐ Mod. ☐ Severe
Description: _____ Frequency:_____ ☐ AM ☐ PM
Radiation: _____ Duration:_____

Secondary Complaint_____ Degree: ☐ Mild ☐ Mod. ☐ Severe
Description: _____ Frequency:_____ ☐ AM ☐ PM
Radiation: _____ Duration:_____

Tertiary Complaint_____ Degree: ☐ Mild ☐ Mod. ☐ Severe
Description: _____ Frequency:_____ ☐ AM ☐ PM
Radiation: _____ Duration:_____

Duration Of Symptoms

First Noticed:_____ ☐ Worse ☐ Improving ☐ Same
Cause:_____
Previous Occurances: ☐ Yes ☐ No Last Occurrence:_____ Frequency:_____

Injuries, Accidents & Stress

☐ Difficult Delivery ☐ Caesarean ☐ Breach ☐ Forceps ☐ Other:_____
☐ Accidents:_____ ☐ Falls:_____
☐ Broken Bones:_____ ☐ Surgeries:_____
☐ Mental Stress:_____ ☐ Physical Stress:_____
☐ Work Stress:_____ ☐ Home Stress:_____

Previous or Other Doctors

This Complaint:_____ When:_____
Different Complaint:_____ When:_____

Tests, Opinions, & Advice

Testing Procedures:_____ When:_____
Opinion or Diagnosis:_____
Recommendations:_____ Compliance:_____

Previous Care & Procedures

Chiropractic: ☐ Yes ☐ No Describe:_____ Results:_____
Medicines: ☐ Yes ☐ No Describe:_____ Results:_____
Phys. Therapy: ☐ Yes ☐ No Describe:_____ Results:_____
Surgery: ☐ Yes ☐ No Describe:_____ Results:_____
Other: ☐ Yes ☐ No Describe:_____ Results:_____

Environmental Links

Job Activities:_____
Hobbies / Sports:_____
Children: Boys:____ Girls:____ Ages:_____ Grandchildren:_____
Sleep Positions: ☐ Side ☐ Back ☐ Stomach Mattress:_____ Pillow:_____
Aggravation From Above:_____

Affect On Lifestyle

Missed Work: ☐ Yes ☐ No When:_____ Restricted Work Activities:_____
Restricted Daily Activities: ☐ Yes ☐ No Explain:_____
Interfere With Sleep: ☐ Yes ☐ No Why:_____
Other:_____

Hereditary

Similar Condition In Family: : ☐ Yes ☐ No Who:_____ What:_____

Other

Sample Form: **New Patient Consultation Worksheet**

plaint? Does the pain radiate? Is the problem constant or does it come and go? If it is intermittent, how frequent is it, and how long does it last? Is it worse in the morning, in the evening, or at night? Does it prevent sleep? And so forth. All of these factors will give the examiner valuable insight into the nature of the patient's possible subluxation complex and its effect on the patient's life.

Of course it is necessary for you to gather this information from an analytical and clinical point of view, but it is also vital for future interaction with a host of other entities. Whether you accept insurance or not, the insurance companies will require such information about their policyholders. Without obtaining this information, it is impossible to properly monitor the patient's progress and assess the effectiveness of care. Most importantly, a complete consultation can be of tremendous value should some future malpractice allegation arise. (I have known more than one doctor who has received notification of an allegation that his or her care has caused a patient's specific complaint, only to have the allegations dismissed because the doctor had properly documented that the patient actually presented with the same complaint.)

It has been said that 80 percent of a doctor's diagnosis is derived from the patient's consultation and history. In fact, most experienced practitioners will usually have a good idea simply from the consultation whether or not they can help the patient, as well as what should be done during the rest of the patient's analytical work-up. An in-depth consultation may ultimately save you time and energy, and save the patient money and discomfort by eliminating unnecessary testing procedures, or the acceptance of a patient who should have been referred.

2. Duration of Symptoms. Determining a causative factor and the chronicity of the patient's complaint is mandatory to determining proper case management. Some patients' problems may be new and acute, while others may have lived with their problems for many years, yet both may present with identical subjective complaints. Obviously, knowing the duration of the patient's symptoms will be crucial as you consider how you will manage both cases.

Some patients may have had multiple injuries that have complicated their problems with layers of accumulated biomechanical stress and trauma, others will present with a new injury that is rather straightforward and easy to understand. Either way, as a clinician, you must understand whether this acute condition for which they are seeing you is a new problem or an acute manifestation of a chronic condition. During the consultation, you may learn that some patients have acute episodes only at certain times of the year. If you can isolate their activities during this time, it might assist you with your evaluation, recommendations, and future clinical management.

Strangely, you will find it is actually uncommon for the average patient to be able to tell you what caused the situation that brought them into your office. Frequently, it is the accumulation of the microtrauma caused by their work habits or lifestyles that caused the gradual breakdown of the spinal integrity. Only with a thorough and detailed consultation can you even begin to understand the true clinical picture and the causative agents of the spinal instabilities and the resultant vertebral subluxations of the new patient.

3. Surgeries or Traumas. Previous episodes of physical stress will have an accumulated impact on the patient's spinal integrity and overall health. Long-ago falls, surgeries, or accidents are subjects that patients will seldom remember to tell you about. Hardly ever will a patient have the insight to connect the fall they had as a child with the headaches that are bringing them to your office many years later. Never do they correlate the stomach surgery they had 10 years ago with their mid-dorsal pain today. And, it's a far stretch of the imagination for the average new patient to link the broken leg they had when they were eight years old with the scoliosis, kidney, or intestinal problems of today.

That is why you must ask your patients about these past incidents. Dig deep into their history of injuries, birth traumas, and past surgical interventions. Be unrelenting in probing the patient's history and insist that these questions are answered completely. Until you do, you will have only a superficial picture of the patient's true clinical condition.

4. Previous Doctors. Unfortunately, too few doctors delve into the patient's treatment history. They do not ask about what other doctors have attempted in an effort to remedy this or any other health concern that the patient may have experienced. Asking one simple question ("What other doctors have you seen in the past five years?") may reveal a laundry list of doctors who have not found the cause of the patient's condition, who did not help the person adjust their lifestyle, doctors who may have merely treated symptoms, others who did not explain their recommendations, and others who simply did not properly manage the patient. Many times, you will get an unsolicited report on the virtues and downfalls of other practitioners. Listen and learn.

5. Testing, Opinions, and Procedures. Just as important as knowing whom the patient has seen in the past, is to learn what has actually been recommended and done for the patient. (By the very nature of the person's being in your office, you will learn what did *not* work.) Also, knowing what examinations and testing procedures were utilized in the past, and what has been ruled out, can be helpful information.

Further insight can be gained by asking the patient about previous doctors' opinions or diagnoses. I have found that a large number of patients who sought my care were doing so simply because previous doctors never reported their findings to the patient, offered an opinion, or explained the rationale for recommended care. (They probably did not perform an adequate consultation either.)

Finally, it is to the patient's benefit for you to know what the previous doctors recommended. Did they advise lifestyle changes that the patient failed to comply with? Did they recommend a specific course of care? Did the patient follow those recommendations? If not, why not? This information will also give you valuable insight into how well the patient may comply with your recommendations.

6. Previous Procedures. Next, you need to know the patient's history of previous treatment, medications, and surgical procedures. It is important that you know what kind of drugs or medications the patient is currently taking. In fact, asking the patient about the frequency of care, duration of care, and the results they attained can give you insight into the severity and chronicity of the patient's condition. An even greater advantage to taking this kind of history is the likelihood of discovering drug abuse, overdose, adverse reactions, or interaction with other drugs that previous doctors may have overlooked.

It is also surprising how many patients try to self-medicate or self-manipulate their spines. It is important that you know just what they have done and are doing. For instance, many patients routinely use heat on painful areas. Although they are probably enhancing the pain, edema, and inflammation, they usually don't tell you they are taking such measures unless specifically asked. (More than once, I have failed to get the results I anticipated with a patient, only to later find that the person had been sleeping with a heating pad or taking drugs of which I was not aware.)

Another necessary question to be asked during the consultation is if the patient has had any previous surgeries. As we know, but patients are seldom told, any surgical procedure structurally and functionally alters the body. You need to know what surgeries were performed before rendering an opinion, giving a prognosis, or commencing care.

7. Environmental Links. Luckily, a little digging into a patient's lifestyle, work requirements, and family history will usually present a picture of the causative factors in the patient's condition (especially if they are biomechanical in nature). Wouldn't this knowledge have a major impact on both your management and prognosis of this patient's case? In our industrialized and sedentary society, many cases we see are directly attributed to patient environmental factors, and without modifying these activities, lasting results may never be attained.

A doctor cannot properly care for a patient without knowing what the person does all day long. Repetitive movements seen in many of today's occupations eventually cause wear and tear on the body, breaking down its supportive structures. Although this is not intended to be a course in ergonomics, the interested, concerned, competent doctor will question the patient's work requirements in-depth and counsel accordingly.

Just as it is important to know what patients do all day at work, you need to be aware of the patient's hobbies and sports activities. Any necessary activity modification by the doctor may mean the difference in failure or success when correcting the patient's subluxation, structural instability, and returning the patient to health.

Also, don't forget that the number of children the patient has borne may directly influence the physical condition of the patient. Likewise, if the patient has children or grandchildren they are caring for, they may be involved in many activities that stress the various structural and soft tissue components of the body. (Not to mention the degree of mental and emotional stress that may affect the severity of their condition or their response to care.) Of great significance also are the ages of the children. Younger children produce a completely different set of physical and mental stressors on their patients than older children.

8. Effect on Lifestyle. As stated previously, new patients seek your care primarily because their physical problems are affecting their ability to work productively or to live the pain-free and abundant life they desire. Asking the patient about the impact of the complaint on their ability to perform the activities they want to do, will give insight into the severity of the complaint, as well as how motivated the patient might be to follow your recommendations and get well.

Here, also, is where you will learn what factors actually motivated this patient to seek your care. The concerned doctor will discuss these influences with the patient and get a clear picture of just how this problem is affecting the person's life. Later, such information may be used as a strong motivator in encouraging the patient to act in his or her own best interest by following through with your recommendations. It will serve as a gauge of how much progress has been achieved.

9. Hereditary Possibilities. Last, what if the patient's condition was caused by an underlying hereditary factor? Would this factor influence the way you approach this case? Certainly, an underlying inherited weakness or structural defect could affect your recommendations, your clinical chiropractic approach to this patient, and ultimately your prognosis for this patient's future recovery. By asking and following up on any genetic patterns of weakness, you will certainly increase your understanding of this patient in a much more profound way.

Predispositions for similar genetic weaknesses may affect the patient's extended family as well as their offspring on either a clinical or subclinical level. By providing such insights, conscientious questioning in the realm of similar health problems in the patient's family may offer an opportunity to serve other family members in a corrective or preventative manner. In addition, such attention to hereditary detail could become the basis for a significant source of referrals either to your practice or to chiropractic in general.

The Patient's First Real Impression of the Doctor

If it is true that the patient's first impressions are formed during the first few minutes of meeting a new doctor, it is then the consultation where the doctor-patient relationships are usually established. This first meeting should always leave patients with an overwhelming confidence that you are thorough, competent, and caring. As their doctor, your ability to influence the patient to the point where they will allow you to care for them in the best manner indicated is totally dependent on the patient's first impression.

As such, the consultation is a huge factor in setting the stage for success or failure in every case. Whether or not the patient accepts you as his or her doctor, adheres to your recommendations, follows through with care, and ultimately acts in his or her own best interest by giving you the opportunity to enhance his or her health and life, are all totally dependent upon the first 15 minutes that you and your patient are together—the consultation.

Step 5-7: Letting Them Know That You Know—the Examination

For many of the same reasons that we recommend our doctors always perform comprehensive consultations, we also strongly recommend that concise, yet comprehensive, examinations be performed on every new patient.

Remember, above all, the patient needs to *know* that you *know*. They want to feel that their doctor has left no "bone unturned" in trying to find out what is wrong. Over the years, I have come to see the examination process as one of the best patient management tools and referral generating procedures there is. Hundreds of patients have been referred to my practice with the words: "Go see Dr. Meyer. He does a great examination and will find your problem."

The examination process is your greatest opportunity to "wow" new patients. This is your chance to actually show you are thorough, knowledgeable, and clinically proficient and that you care about your patients to the point that you always go the extra mile. The ultimate compliment a patient can give a doctor is to tell others, "That doctor gave me the best examination I ever had." Translated: "This doctor is sharp and really knows his or her business." In short, give the new patient the best chiropractic examination possible and they will accept your recommendations for care—and tell others.

Establishing Systems for a Smooth First Visit

When performing a new patient examination, always begin at the patient's primary complaint. Before you do anything else, palpate the spot where the patient tells you it hurts. If it is their hand, palpate their hand. If it is their head, palpate their head. If the complaint is abdominal, palpate the abdomen. The main reason for this practice is that it tells the patient you know where they hurt, you understand their symptoms, and you were listening during the consultation.

Even when we, as chiropractors, know that the pain in the patient's shoulder is probably coming from the neck, the patient does not understand it—*yet*. More than once, I have ignored my own procedure and gone directly to the spine on a new patient, only to have the patient get frustrated and tell me all over again where the symptom actually is. Believe me—it is easier and faster to demonstrate to patients that you know where they hurt by checking that area first.

Also, it is a good habit to x-ray the patient at the point of pain, in addition to the corresponding spinal areas that you normally would x-ray. Otherwise, the patient will always wonder if you missed something (and maybe you will too!).

Several years ago, a young man entered my office with complaints of neck and shoulder pain. An examination of the cervical spine revealed numerous findings that led me to conclude the shoulder complaints were stemming from the neck and a resulting irritation of the brachial plexus. Much to my surprise, a simple a-p view of the shoulder revealed an osteosarcoma on the head of the humerus. You never know what you might find. That one-in-a-million lesion you discover could make you a hero, not to mention possibly saving your professional reputation as well as your practice.

Another major benefit to palpating and x-raying the area of the patient's complaint is that when you have demonstrated there is nothing wrong with the area of pain, you have the confidence and authority to sit down with the patient and tell him or her that "even though you may have pain in your leg, nothing is wrong with your leg." This statement then sets the stage for the patient to understand the chiropractic concept of nerve impingement, referred pain, and how deceiving and clinically unimportant most symptoms can actually be.

As was mentioned earlier, the examination is second only to the consultation in building a strong doctor-patient relationship. While you may not lose a patient through a shoddy examination, you will have certainly lost an important tool to manage that patient. The degree of thoroughness in your examination is in direct proportion to the degree of acceptance and follow-through you will receive from the patient.

While performing the examination, it is extremely helpful for the examiner to purposefully explain to the patient what each test is designed to show. Then, when positive indications are discovered, the examiner should stop and explain how these findings relate to the patient's actual complaint. By the time you are finished with the examination (if done properly), your patient should be at the point of having an elementary understanding as to what is causing the problem. Wouldn't it be great to be able to complete the examination and have the patient say, "Gee, doc, it sounds like I have 'disc bulge,' 'muscle spasm,' and 'nerve interference.' Just what do you think is causing all this?" And you can then say, "Mrs. Jones, you may have a subluxated vertebra in your spine; let's take some x-rays of your spine and see if we can find it."

In most instances, strong indications for the presence of the various components of a vertebral subluxation can be observed and documented by a proper examination. Such findings will then naturally lead to an effective case consultation in which you only need to restate, clarify, and reinforce what the patient has already learned during the examination.

Transition Statement Two: The Pre-Examination

After completing the consultation, you should take a few moments and mentally review all of the information that was developed in this process. Quite often, you will want to orally review your notes so that the patient understands just how thorough the consultation actually was. Once you have finished reviewing the consultation, you should again look the patient straight in the eye and deliver the next statement that will effectively transition the patient to the examination:

> **Doctor:** "Mrs. Jones, is there anything I should have asked or that you would like to know that we did not cover before we go on?
>
> "If not, our next step is try to discover the true underlying cause of your complaints. To do this, I would like to examine your entire spine and nerve system. Also, we need to see if there are any other

Establishing Systems for a Smooth First Visit

problems that may be developing as a result of: (list any previous falls, accidents, or injuries that were discussed during the consultation).

"If I can find the cause of your problem and I feel I can help you, I will. But, if not, I will tell you that right away and I will help you to find someone who might.

"Do you have any questions?"

By asking the patient if they "have any questions," you will be giving them the opportunity to present any hesitation or fears they may have. When the patient reports there are no questions, they are giving you tacit permission to continue. Such an opportunity will prevent the patient from feeling they are being "railroaded" and that you are pressuring the them to continue.

The Examination Process

A good entrance examination has many aspects. Before we discuss the various individual tests and their indications, let's discuss their sequence. As you begin, you must consider that you are moving the patient from the consultative position of sitting into a new and different position for the examination. I recommend that you begin the exam by palpating the patient's area of complaint, then placing the patient in a sitting position. Sitting is generally an easier position for the patient to assume initially, and it does not place the patient in the more submissive prone or supine position. Generally, having the patient sit on the edge of the exam table is best. I recommend you perform all of the basic physical checks that can be done in this position.

Besides the obvious clinical value of performing a good examination, it is just as important that you demonstrate your thoroughness and competence. A concise, yet thorough, examination will reinforce the possibility of any enduring spinal or neurological limitations that may have been caused by long-ago injuries. The examination should also help the doctor to confirm or rule out his or her initial clinical suspicions formed during the consultation. And finally, the examination should give you an idea as to the appropriateness of a possible referral of this patient.

Subluxation Examination

Patient: _____ Date: _____ Exam#: _____

Posture & Movement

Postural Analysis
- Head Tilt ☐ Lt ☐ Rt + _____
- Shoulder Tilt ☐ Lt ☐ Rt + _____
- Pelvic Tilt ☐ Lt ☐ Rt + _____

Weight Bearing
- Weight: _____
- Distr: ☐ Lt ☐ Rt + _____
- Stability: _____

Lumbar Range of Motion

	Degrees	Pain
Flex Ion	___/90	___
Extension	___/45	___
L. Rot	___/30	___
R. Rot	___/30	___
L. Flex	___/30	___
R. Flex	___/30	___

Cervical Range of Motion

	Degrees	Pain
Flex Ion	___/45	___
Extension	___/45	___
L. Rot	___/80	___
R. Rot	___/80	___
L. Flex	___/45	___
R. Flex	___/45	___

Nerve System

Reflexes

	Lt.	Rt.
Biceps	___	___
Triceps	___	___
Extensors	___	___
Patellar	___	___
Achilles	___	___

Neuro-Ortho Testing
- For Comp _____
- Max Comp _____
- Sh Dep _____
- Distract _____
- Valsalva _____

- Cranial Nerves: _____
- Dermatomes: _____
- Kemp's Sign _____
- Toe Walk _____
- Heel Walk _____
- Rhomberg: _____
- Other: _____

Muscle & Strength

Circumference

	Lt.	Rt.
Thigh	___	___
Calve	___	___
Biceps	___	___
Forearm	___	___

Neuro-Ortho Testing
- SotoHall: _____
- S.L.R: _____
- Braggard: _____
- Leg Drop: _____

Dynamometer
- Lt Hand _____
- Rt Hand _____

Vitals
- Blood Pressure:
  - Lt _____
  - Rt _____
- VBA: _____
- Subclavian: _____
- Carotid: _____
- Heart: _____

Palpatory Examination

	LMS	LTP	SP	RTP	RMS
OC					
C1					
C2					
C3					
C4					
C5					
C6					
C7					
T1					
T2					
T3					
T4					
T5					
T6					
T7					
T8					
T9					
T10					
T11					
T12					
L1					
L2					
L3					
L4					
L5					

SACRUM

Sample Form: **Subluxation Examination**

In any examination sequence, patients always expect to have their blood pressure taken. It is advantageous to do this at the start for several reasons. First, following the consultation, the patient may be more at ease, so your readings may be more accurate than after having the patient move through the other procedures. More importantly, obtaining bilateral blood pressure readings is a major factor in performing George's Cerebral-Vascular Test. Following bilateral blood pressure, the examiner should then ausculate the subclavian and carotid arteries, and perform a vertebral-basilar artery function assessment. By performing these procedures, you know immediately whether or not you have a high-risk (stroke) patient and how to proceed with the rest of the examination.

With the patient still sitting and with the examiner still holding the stethoscope, the exam naturally flows into a quick check of the lung and heart sounds. In a chiropractic practice this is not done to render any diagnosis for these organs, but merely to rule out the presence of any abnormalities that may, again, require a referential decision. The examiner can then look for any abnormalities in the eyes, ears, nose, and throat without moving the patient, followed by cranial nerve testing, and a quick check of any dermatome that may appear to be involved.

Finally, you should test the patient's reflexes in both the arms and the legs; grip strength; and circumference measurements of the thigh, calve, biceps, and forearm. At this point, the patient often will remark as to your thoroughness or the fact that no one has ever checked these areas before. Little does the patient know that this is just the beginning of a complete chiropractic examination process.

Now, with the patient still sitting, the examiner can move naturally into testing the cervical ranges of motion (kinesiopathology) and various orthopedic tests such as the Foramina Compression Test, Maximum Cervical Compression, Shoulder Depression, Cervical Distraction, Valsalva's Maneuver, or any other seated exam the practitioner wishes.

Once all of the seated testing is completed, the patient should be placed in the prone position on the examination table for spinal palpation assessment and the other various procedures that you determine necessary. In offices where no instrumentation is used, the examination and recording procedures examination can serve as a fundamental assessment of the spine. By grading each segmental level (1 through 5) in a graphic manner, you can subjectively quantify and record the degree of muscle spasm (MS) (myopathophysiology), trigger points (TP) (neuropathophysiology), and spinous process (SP) tenderness (histopathology/ligamentous degeneration). Then, you can subjectively rate and record these findings to be used as comparisons later. Such an examination, if performed and recorded with care and diligence, can later be a major asset in comparative reevaluation and effective patient management throughout all three stages of condition-based care.

Then, the patient may be instructed to turn over onto their back for the necessary supine tests such as Soto-Hall's Test, Linder's Test, SLR, Braggard's Sign, Goldthwait, Gaenslen's, etc. Once completed in this position, the patient can be stood erect where the lumbar ranges of motion (spinopathokinesiolgy) can be measured. Such tests as Kemp's, Lewin's Punch Test, Trendelenburg's, Rhomberg's, and the toe and heel walk should also be considered.

Upon completion of these various standing tests, the patient can be analyzed posturally and weight bearing measured on dual scales. Use of a posture-analyzing device can be a great visual tool in showing the patient the structural inconsistencies in their posture. A quick review of any postural distortions or weight-bearing discrepancies creates an instinctive transition to the radiological examination.

> *Note:* Although this examination is thorough and comprehensive in exhibiting numerous components of the subluxation, you should remember that the more time-consuming aspects of the tests, notably those tests where the results are objectively measurable, may be performed by a competent and well-trained CA. Therefore, the CA may perform such procedures as the circumferential measurements, range of motion (if a goniometer is used), postural analysis, and vitals. As a matter of prudence, it is recommend that the doctor review these findings and recheck anything suspicious. Of course, the parts of the examination that require professional judgment and interpretation should only be performed by the doctor.

Conclusion

The above testing procedures, when laid out in a concise logical format, should flow so naturally and efficiently that it requires little wasted time moving the patient between positions. Although such a procedure can be performed in 12 to 15 minutes, the patient's concept is that of having just experienced an in-depth, complete examination of all of the major areas in question.

All of the tests, signs, and observations included in the examination are designed to do three specific things. First, they aid you in arriving at an accurate impression of the patient's problem. Second, they help to indicate the presence of the vertebral subluxation based upon the presence of the physical effects of the subluxation complex. Third, they give you and the patient an objective assessment of the presenting problem and an objective measurement of the patient's response to care. These tests all fall into four categories that demonstrate specific entities usually found in the presence of the vertebral subluxation:

1. The involvement of nerve tissue and the disturbance of the trophic and functional aspects of the nervous system.
2. The presence of spinal imbalance, vertebral fixation, and postural distortion.
3. The effect of the muscular adaptation from the nerve impingement or the postural distortion.
4. The presence of strain/sprain type effects of the soft tissue surrounding the offending vertebral segment.

The examination process is specifically designed to locate, document, and monitor the presence and effects of the vertebral subluxations. The only procedures that are not mentioned here are those specific to your particular technique analysis and the use of thermographic instrumentation to monitor the physiological effect of the vertebral subluxation on the skin surface temperature, surface EMGs, or the use of other such instruments as the various functional recording and analysis systems that are becoming increasingly popular in detecting the various components of the Vertebral Subluxation Complex. Such instrumentation procedures are highly recommended for understanding the patient and for the patient's understanding of chiropractic. In addition, they will enhance the development of the doctor-patient relationship, eventually leading to the patient accepting your recommendations and follow-through with needed care and long-term management of the patient.

The real value to this exam is that it brings to the patient a chiropractic awareness of the objectification of the damaging effects of the vertebral subluxations. That is why I cannot emphasize strongly enough the extreme importance of a good examination. While performing the examination, it is imperative that you explain the findings and consequences of each individual positive test as it is performed. Relating each examination finding to the nervous system and the spine is the most effective and efficient patient education tool available to you. A large amount of chiropractic enlightenment can be produced within the patient simply by briefly describing the test, the findings, and the clinical significance as they are performed and experienced by the patient.

Finally, the exam should always move along quickly and with a high degree of emphasis given to each test and each positive finding. The conclusions the patient may draw from your descriptive examination form the first and most important step in the patient's understanding of the Vertebral Subluxation Complex and its crucial implications for their health.

Finally, the gross postural analysis of the patient is extremely important for the patient to visualize the postural distortions and adaptations that may have taken place. There are several posture analyzing tools on the market that will both demonstrate and objectify the postural distortions patients will present. However, the use of a full-length wall mirror that has been taped off with a centerline plus shoulder and pelvic lines allows the patient to see for themselves their postural deviations, and will greatly enhance your ability to demonstrate any postural aberrations to the patient. As with every other positive examination, each abnormality, its consequences, and probable cause should be verbally noted and reinforced to the patient. Once this procedure has been completed and the distortions recorded, the patient is ready to progress to the x-ray phase of the exam.

Step 5-8 : Seeing Is Believing and Understanding—X-Raying the New Patient

After the exam is completed and the patient is seated, the doctor should sit on the edge of the table and discuss with the patient the possible need for an x-ray examination. The radiological exam of the patient's spine is a vital tool, allowing you to analyze the patient's vertebral subluxation complex and the actual condition of the spine and the corresponding structures.

The films also serve as an effective educational tool that will enhance the patient's understanding of their vertebral subluxation and its health implications. High quality x-rays also give you the ability to understand the degree of subluxation degeneration that has occurred. Such an understanding will logically and inevitably lead to accurate case recommendations and an improved ability to give the patient an informed prognosis of his or her response to care.

This transition from the examination to the recommending of appropriate films is often difficult for some doctors, usually a result of the doctor's fear of rejection because of the cost of the procedure to the patient or other patient concerns. If, however, everything is performed exactly as described to this point, seldom (if ever) will a doctor encounter any resistance to having radiological studies performed.

Transition Statement Three: Post-Exam/Pre X-Ray Statement

This particular transition statement is vital because it not only transitions the patient to the x-ray process, but it restates the examination findings in a concise manner. If you properly described the findings during the examination, this statement will reinforce in the patient's mind just what the problems truly are. By doing this, you are laying the basis for an effective and well-accepted case review on the following day.

> **Doctor:** "Mrs. Jones, it appears that your problems are being caused by an involvement of the nerves, disc, (review exam results) etc. in this area of your spine (doctor touching area). Your previous history of (falls, accidents, or injuries) has probably caused or at least contributed to these findings.
>
> "We have a good idea of the spinal structures involved, and where your complaints are stemming from. But we cannot know from the exam what may actually be causing them. Nor do we know the extent of the damage or how your body has tried to heal in this area.
>
> "To determine that, we will need to take a couple pictures of your spine so we can view these problem areas.
>
> "If you will come with me, it will just take a few minutes and hopefully we can get to the bottom of this."

After making the transition statement, the doctor will simply turn slowly, lead the patient to the x-ray area, and take the necessary films.

Step 5-9: Committed and Concerned— Releasing the New Patient

After the examination and x-rays are completed, it is now necessary to release the new patient. Properly executed, the release will give the patient some indication of the preliminary findings as well as explain to them why no care will be rendered at this initial visit. The release should be done in such a manner as to make the patient aware of the seriousness of the condition, but without unduly alarming them. Properly conceived and delivered with the right intent, it will leave the patient with the feeling that the doctor is competent and caring.

At this point, it is also important to advise the patient of any home measures that may be taken to make the patient as comfortable as possible overnight.

Many doctors find it difficult not to care for the patient on the initial visit. But, to adjust a patient on the initial visit is a serious procedural error that will significantly hamper your ability to successfully lead the patient through the initial relief phase of care and on to true wellness. If you find it difficult not to render some sort of care to the patient, remember that this patient's problem has probably been developing for quite some time and seldom does even the patient expect immediate relief. To adjust the patient on the first visit is usually a result of low personal and professional confidence and ultimately runs many needless risks in patient care and case management. The reasons for this are many:

1. The patient has not had the opportunity to learn about the nature of the problem, the type of care offered, and to consent to such care as an informed patient.

2. Not knowing what the chiropractor is attempting to do during the first adjustment, the patient may be apprehensive and unable to relax. This may make the adjustment painful or even contraindicated.

3. Immediate care may imply immediate relief. When immediate relief is not forthcoming, the patient may judge chiropractic on just one adjustment and immediately discontinue care, feeling that chiropractic has been tried—and failed.

4. On the other hand, if significant relief is effected, the patient may get the impression that chiropractic is a great form of temporary relief, and consequently, never avail themselves of the more beneficial aspects of corrective and wellness care.
5. You may be hurried by the pressing needs of other patients, the desire to keep on schedule, or the desire to shorten the amount of time that the new patient remains in the office. In this haste, you may actually miss something on the x-ray or exam, and thereby perform an ineffective or contraindicated adjustment.

Therefore, only in rare instances should the patient be adjusted on the first visit. Instead, you should release the patient to come back the following day. At the same time, it is necessary that the patient be given a logical reason as to why no actual care will be given that day and an explanation of what to expect on the following visit. Thus, the fourth transition statement—the dismissal—is the most important of all of the transition statements.

Transition Statement Four: The Dismissal

Always remember that the last words you say to the patient will be the most remembered aspect of the entire visit. Therefore, you must choose the right words and leave the patient with the right "feeling" as you deliver the new patient to the front desk. The following is an example of an effective transition statement to use when releasing a new patient:

Doctor: "Mrs. Jones, it will take us a couple of hours to process, analyze, and review your films. Later this evening, I will sit down and study them and correlate them with the information from your consultation, your health history, and your examination findings. Therefore we have done all that we can today.

"When you return tomorrow I will sit down with you and explain exactly what we have discovered—explain the examination results, and show you your x-rays.

"Would it be possible for your husband (spouse) to come with you? I would like him to understand your condition and to know what you have been going through." (Try to get a commitment for the spouse if possible.)

"Let's go up and have Carol arrange an appointment time for you and your husband tomorrow."

At that point, you may simply stand and lead the patient to the front desk. When at the front desk (with the patient listening) you should instruct the CA to reserve enough (additional) time on the proper day for a review of the case and for an adjustment, and at a time when the patient's spouse can attend as well.

These directions should be given to the CA in such a manner that you are actually reinforcing to the patient the appointment should not be taken lightly and should be made at a time when the spouse can attend. As previously discussed, reinforcing to the patient what will be accomplished on the next visit, as well as providing added encouragement for the patient to bring the spouse along, will prepare the patient for the second visit.

Doctor: "Carol, would you find a time tomorrow for Mrs. Jones and her husband? Please set extra time for me to review our findings for her today and to show her x-rays."

Next, you should turn to the patient, placing a hand on the patient's shoulder, and tell the patient you will be ready for them tomorrow. Then turn and leave the front desk area immediately, allowing the front desk CA to do his or her job.

Step 5-10: Successfully Collecting the First Day Fees

If the patient has health insurance that (from previous experience with the carrier, you believe) will cover their services, collection techniques should be minimal. To avoid the appearance of hiding anything from the patient, the front desk CA should review the charges for the first visit and give the patient the opportunity to pay for the day's services. Keep in mind that the first day's collection policies and procedures should absolutely never dampen the patient's enthusiasm for their new doctor, their first visit experience, or the great first impression that has been developing throughout the entire first visit.

Therefore, when the new patient is returned to the front desk, the CA should simply place the completed service slip on the counter in

◆ Establishing Systems for a Smooth First Visit ◆

front of the patient and point to each individual service that was performed and say:

CA: "Mrs. Jones, your charges for today are $50 for the consultation and the examination and $99 for the x-ray study. Besides cash or check, we also accept Visa and MasterCard."

If the patient hesitates or can only make a partial payment, the CA should be gracious and inform the patient that specific arrangements will be made on the next visit:

CA: "I understand, Mrs. Jones. I will call your insurance company this afternoon, to check your coverage. I will review it with you tomorrow and we will set up some arrangements then."

It is important to remember that the patient has just enjoyed a wonderful experience in your office. They have found a caring and efficient staff. They just received a thorough consultation and had a comprehensive examination by a doctor who is warm, compassionate, and highly competent. The front desk, within view of other patients, is *not* the time to undo all this goodwill by utilizing heavy-handed collection techniques.

When the patient leaves your office after the first visit, your goal is to have them on "cloud nine." Your collection policies, procedures, and staff must be designed, developed, and taught to not cause the new patient to start having any doubts about their ability to receive the care they need and to enjoy the benefits of being cared for in your office. The last thing we want them to be concerned with is money. Financial arrangements will be more easily made on the second visit, behind closed doors, after the case review, with the patient fully understanding their case and their doctor's recommendations.

Step 5-11: Scheduling the Second Appointment/Spouse at Report

After collecting the first day's fees, the CA will naturally move to scheduling the patient's next appointment. For the second visit, time will be reserved for you to review the case with the patient, as well as for the patient to be adjusted. Approximately 30 minutes should be reserved for this visit.

It is also important that the CA attempt to follow the doctor's orders and that a concerted effort be made to get the patient's spouse to attend the case review. Therefore, in scheduling the second appointment the CA should emphasize the spouse's schedule, not just the patient's

> **CA:** "Mrs. Jones, tomorrow the doctor will discuss with you what (he or she) has found, and give you an idea of what will be necessary to properly address your health concerns. The doctor feels it is important that Mr. Jones attends also so that he can understand what you have been going through. Which would be better for him tomorrow? Morning or afternoon? Early or late?"

Releasing the New Patient

After the payment procedures have been handled and the new appointment made, the CA will thank the patient and tell them again how pleased he or she is that the patient has chosen your practice and he or she should reaffirm that the doctor will be ready for them at the appointed time.

A proper release of the patient by both the doctor and the CA is important for these reasons. First, a proper release justifies the fact that the patient is not being adjusted that day. Second, it also helps the patient see the possible seriousness of their health concerns. Third, it gives them an idea of what to expect on the next visit.

Step 5-12: Committing a Procedural Error Adjusting on the First Visit

Adjusting the patient on the first visit always presents some serious procedural problems that may produce several unforeseen adverse consequences. Very seldom, and only in cases of extreme emergencies, should a patient be adjusted on the first day and even more seldom on the first visit.

The major concern with adjusting the patient on the first visit is that it tends to imply immediate relief of the patient's presenting pain or other symptoms, which ultimately may lead to unrealistic expectations of you and of chiropractic. Then, if immediate relief is not forthcoming, it may lead to doubts about the effectiveness of chiropractic and the doctor. Without the time to digest what has been done on the first visit, without the benefit of the case review and the ability to make an informed decision to proceed with care, the patient has no real concept of what you have done to them or what to expect in the future. In instances where expectations are not met and immediate relief not effected (or even in cases where symptomatic relief exceeds expectations) unchanged perceptions of chiropractic care may prevent the patient from understanding the real objectives of chiropractic, causing them to be destined to a live a subluxated, unfulfilled life of pain, illness, or simply a lack of innate health.

From a legal point of view, taking shortcuts and rushing a patient through the first visit leaves the impression that you were not thorough. In fact, an uneducated patient receiving an adjustment without proper explanation may even feel assaulted and battered by the initial adjustment, leading to many more problems down the road.

Most importantly, the patients must be allowed to become informed, to participate in, and to make an educated decision about the course of their own healthcare. Without taking the time needed to describe the subluxation complex and its ramifications, the rationale for care, and explaining your recommendations for successful correction of the presenting subluxations, your patient is simply not able to make an educated decision regarding your recommendations or the utilization of chiropractic to enhance their future level of wellness.

That being said, on occasions, special circumstances may exist where you may feel it necessary to attempt to afford the patient some relief on the first day. This situation may also occur when x-rays are not taken and you may not be able to justify taking the extra time. In such situations, I recommend that the patient be sent out of the office for a few hours allowing you to study, digest, and ponder the patient's case and decide on a deliberate course of action. This precaution also gives the patient time to reflect on the thoroughness of the consultation and examination process they have just experienced.

Anytime a patient is adjusted on the first visit with or without x-rays, you must take special precautions to explain exactly what is being done before, during, and after adjusting the patient. The following is a script that may be used when adjusting on the first visit with or without x-rays. Study it, learn it, and use it sparingly.

Doctor: "Mrs. Jones, what we are seeing is a situation where there is pressure on your spinal nerves, some disc involvement, and a lot of muscle spasm (components of VSC). These are all being caused by a misalignment of one or more of the vertebrae in your spine that can be seen on your x-rays.

"I would like to begin the process of correcting this problem right away. But I want you to understand you may experience little actual relief today. That is because we are going to work to correct the cause of your condition, not simply 'treat' your symptoms. Then, tomorrow, we will sit down and I will explain everything to you and your spouse.

"Do you have any questions before we begin?"

At this point, the doctor may help the patient onto the adjusting table by placing one hand on her middle back and verbally directing the patient in the proper way to get on the table

Doctor: "As I mentioned during the exam, your nerves are being pinched by this spinal bone right here (palpate level of subluxation) that is slightly misaligned. This is what is causing your (name symptoms or complaints). I am going to begin the process of adjusting these hard bones away from the delicate nerves along your spine. When I do, you will hear a slight popping sound as the vertebrae shift. It will not hurt and I will be as gentle as possible.

"Do you have any questions?"

Again, by continually asking the patients for questions and addressing their concerns at each point of transition in their care, you will effect tacit permission to proceed and the first adjustment may be given.

Delivering the Patient's First Adjustment

It is extremely important that the patient's first adjustment is given as gently as possible and that it causes no discomfort. Keep in mind that the patient is always somewhat apprehensive and therefore tense prior to their first adjustment. This apprehension naturally raises the likelihood that the initial adjustment will not be as easy on you or the patient as subsequent adjustments. Understanding this, you must never try to do too much. And never, ever cause the patient any discomfort with the adjustment. Especially when the patient is being adjusted on the first visit, it is always better to do too little than too much. With a proper explanation of the situation, and the adjustment procedure, the patient will be better relaxed and not have unrealistic expectations of immediate results. Such an understanding will help take the pressure off and allow you to not try to do too much on the first visit.

Transition Statement Five: The Post-Adjustment Release

After the initial adjustment, whether on the first or the second visit, it is important to sum up the entire experience for the patient and to tell them what you have just done and what immediate results they may expect. At this point, the patient is likely to be overwhelmed by everything they have learned on that visit and by the adjustment. Therefore, to be effective this transition statement must be as simple and direct as possible. At the same time you must speak in a low, relaxed, reassuring manner so that the relaxation process initiated by the adjustment is not compromised.

Doctor: "Okay, Mrs. Jones, we have begun the process of correcting the underlying cause of your problems. You will need to have that adjusted again tomorrow."

Conclusion

We all are given to first impressions of things, occurrences, and experiences in our lives. First impressions are both strong and lasting. Creating a wonderful impression of your practice, your procedures, and your skills is the first step in creating a lifelong wellness patient for your practice.

Always keep in mind that every policy, procedure, word, touch, and smile are being analyzed and interpreted by the patient. Combine friendliness, confidence, thoroughness, and clinical excellence, and the patient will know yours is a quality practice. This is how you begin to build your dream practice—on the first visit with the first patient and their first impression.

Key Points

- The CA's ultimate success in booking the new patient is completely dependent upon answering the patient's specific questions effectively.
- Changing the patient's impression of your practice from a "doctor's office" to "a special place of love and professionalism" will set the stage for many wonderful results.
- Group or personal health insurance coverage should never be taken for granted.
- By asking patients if they "have any questions," you are giving them the opportunity to reveal any hesitation or fears they may have.
- The first day's collection policies and procedures should be designed to never dampen the patient's enthusiasm or the great first impression that has been developing throughout the entire first visit.
- The real value of the exam is to cause a dawning of chiropractic (awareness in the patient).
- To adjust a patient on the initial visit is a serious procedural error that will significantly hamper your ability to successfully lead the patient through the initial relief phase of care and on to true wellness
- Always remember that the last words you say to the patient will be the most remembered aspect of the entire visit.
- Especially when the patient is being adjusted on the first visit, it is always better to do too little than too much.

Solution 6

Create Lifelong Chiropractic Patients

Prior to the return of the new patient for their second visit, a significant amount of activity by both the doctor and the CA must take place. In fact, here more than in any other situation, teamwork between the doctor and the staff is vitally important. Both must be prepared for the patient's second visit. Executed properly, the second visit will be the launching pad for a long and beneficial relationship with your office.

Before the patient's second visit, all preparation, decisions, and communications between the doctor and staff regarding the management of the patient must be completed. Not being organized and prepared for the patient when he or she returns can be disastrous for the patient, their health, and their future. If the doctor and staff are not prepared, it will soon become evident to the patient. Being mentally, emotionally, and organizationally prepared is something that cannot be faked. The patient will sense it immediately.

First, all of the x-ray studies that were taken on the initial visit must be developed and analyzed, and all x-ray listings recorded on the patient information card. At this point, the doctor should have made a diagnosis and have it, too, recorded on the patient information card. In addition, the doctor should also have correlated all examination and x-ray data and arrived at a decision on how to proceed with the case, and what kind of case (visit frequency) recommendations will be made to the patient.

As we now know, the Palmer "Triangle of Care" is an extremely comprehensive and valuable model of chiropractic care that doctors, staff, and even patients understand and readily accept. It represents the big picture of quality chiropractic management of the patient. Although your dream practice may exist inside only one of these three areas of patient care, for the majority of doctors, the practice of their dreams represents a portion of each of these types of patients. In fact, the three types of patient care described in the "Palmer Triangle" probably best represents a successful and maturing practice.

If you are overhauling an existing practice, the best plan of action is to begin with the patients you presently have no matter what phase of care they may be in, and begin to properly educate them as to the benefits of a chiropractic lifestyle and lifelong care. A new practice, of course, will be made up primarily of patients who have come to your office for the relief of symptoms and the complications of an active Vertebral Subluxation Complex. In other words, your practice is, or will initially be, full of patients seeking and receiving condition-based care. Such patients will require you to analyze their case for the potential causes of their presenting complaints and to determine the management that may be most appropriate in their care. Initially, these patients require a rather intensive initial course of care; therefore, special policies, procedures, and considerations must be made in managing their clinical, financial, and educational needs. The time you spend with these patients is valuable and must be used productively in educating and developing healthcare and wellness-care conscientiousness.

Effectively designed, these policies and procedures will set the stage for each new patient to understand chiropractic and make the ultimate decision to become a lifelong chiropractic patient. Thereby, they will avail themselves of the tremendous health and wellness potential generated through comprehensive chiropractic management.

The ultimate focus of educating and developing these patients into individuals who have a true understanding of the long-term benefits of chiropractic should be the basis of every activity in your day-to-day patient interaction. Building your proactive practice requires that it be filled with individuals who ultimately understand chiropractic's beneficial impact on their optimal function and their ability to adapt to internal and external environmental stressors.

It is often during the initial condition-based phase of care that you have both the time and the patient's attention to promote this advanced understanding of chiropractic and its real health-enhancing values. At the same time, swift clinical success is paramount to the doctor enjoying the credibility necessary to change a patient's chiropractic and wellness paradigm. Both strong clinical skills and effective management are enormously essential for this success.

While proper clinical management of this initial phase allows the patient to experience the benefits of subluxation reduction to the greatest extent possible in the shortest period of time, this phase of care will concurrently give the doctor and staff many opportunities to educate the patient on the concepts and benefits of both healthcare and wellness/development care.

For better understanding, as well as simplicity and basic patient management, I have found it advantageous to break down condition-based care into its three primary objectives. The successful realization of the three objectives of will provide the patient with a most successful outcome during this phase. At the same time, such success will set the stage to naturally transition the patient into the more advanced aspects of health and wellness care.

Prior to the delivery of the new patient's case report, you must arrive at a decision as to what recommendations are appropriate to propose to the patient during this early phase of care. Such recommendations will, of course, vary depending on factors that were discovered during the consultation, examination, and x-ray examination. Although each practitioner, depending on skill and technique, may come up with a variable set of recommendations for the patient's initial conditioned-based care, the process of reducing your most common recommendations to a consistent predetermined program will both simplify and expedite the clinical decision-making process, the case management plan, and the making of financial arrangements.

Step 6-1: Provide Objective— Grade-Based Recommendations

Case Recommendations for Initial Intensive Care

Effective case recommendations for initial intensive care consists of making appropriate and reasonable recommendations. These are important in educating patients to understand the rationale for care, and enable them to accept the specific recommendations designed by the doctor. Furthermore, such patients will be more apt to make a successful transition from condition-based care to becoming lifelong chiropractic patients who avail themselves of the best that chiropractic has to offer: lifetime health and wellness care.

During the initial phase of care, success depends on basing all recommendations on specific objectives. At the same time, you must realize every patient is different and that giving the same recommendations to everyone, independent of their clinical presentation of individual circumstances, is intellectually dishonest and clinically indefensible. Depending upon technique, desired outcomes, and the patient's circumstances, you must develop a method of rating each presenting patient in such a way as to be able to quickly and accurately recommend the appropriate level of care. I recommend that, again, based on your technique, skill, and desired outcome, you develop a system similar to the one below. Such a system will allow you to categorize the patient into a level of initial care consistent with the patient's clinical degree of need.

The following is a system similar to the one used in our office for many years. By objectively grading patients into various levels of subjective and objective observations, the patient's level of initial care may quickly and accurately be determined.

Condition-Based Care

A new patient entering the practice usually spends some degree of time receiving condition-based care. As we have already discussed, within this initial phase of care, there are essentially three basic objectives of every case: relief, correction, and stabilization.

Relief Care

The initial phase of patient care is that of providing relief for the symptomatic patient. In most cases, this is achieved by caring for the patient on a rather intensive initial sequence of adjustments designed to reduce the vertebral misalignment until a degree of correction can be effected that will result in a reduction of the patient's presenting symptom complex.

Corrective Care

The primary objective of the second level of condition-based care is to correct, to the greatest degree possible, the misalignment component as well as the accompanying neurological and physiological components of the Vertebral Subluxation Complex. This phase of care is often the most difficult and time-consuming sequence of visits requiring time for the healing of the supporting tissue of the spine, stabilization of neurological function, the long-term restoration of spinal stability, and continual emphasis being placed on the patient's understanding of the corrective purpose of this phase of care. The success of the correction of the clinical aspects of the patient's situation will be based on the clinical findings of the initial subluxation examination and the comparisons of the subsequent progress reevaluations.

Spinal Stabilization

The third objective of initial condition-based care is to ensure that appropriate healing and stabilization has occurred to the point that normal daily activities will not cause a relapse of symptoms or re-subluxation of the patient. This objective may take quite awhile to achieve, but it is generally much less visit frequency intensive as the previous two objectives.

Once each of these objectives has been successfully attained, the patient has usually experienced and understands the true health-enhancing benefits of remaining subluxation-free. This patient will naturally (almost unconsciously) move into a wellness system of long-term care, therefore, joining the ranks of the hundreds of patients who will eventually populate your practice.

Making Recommendations for Condition-Based Care

The following sequences of initial "condition-based care" recommendations are merely examples of the type of recommendations that should be designed based on your techniques, adjusting skills, and experience. Each doctor and each practice will design different frequencies of visits and duration of care. The important thing to remember is that it is vital for you to perform effective initial examinations and frequent reevaluations that will give an accurate picture of the patient's case and their subsequent progress, thereby exhibiting an understanding and a rationale for your case recommendations.

Patient Triage and Objective-Based Recommendations

Prior to determining clinical recommendations for your patients, it is helpful to ascertain where your patient actually falls on the continuum of chronicity, subluxation degeneration, and acuteness of the patient's presenting symptomatology. Judging, or grading the new patient into specific categories based on their subjective and objective status will more easily allow for the subsequent determination and realistic recommendations for a specific course of clinical care.

For simplicity, I have designed three specific categories or grades of new patients. You may find it helpful to develop clinical guidelines for more than these three types of patients. That is fine, in fact, encouraged. The following are descriptions of the three basic categories of cases that we have used for almost thirty years in our private practice. Most patients can easily be placed in one of these three categories, thus allowing for the determination and presentation of accurate and objective case recommendations.

Grade I

The Grade I patient is usually a younger adult or even a child who has no history of trauma or chronic complaints. The initial patient complaint is that of minimal pain, usually restricted to only one area of concern. There is no disability in this case, and the onset is relatively recent with no significant or similar history. There may or may not be a history of trauma. If there is, it is usually minor in the patient's view.

The doctor should always question this patient thoroughly about previous injuries, illnesses, or possible lifestyle stressors. Especially if the presenting patient is an adult, the doctor should delve intently into the above issues to ensure there are no complicating factors or issues the patient may view as insignificant and, therefore, not disclosing to the doctor. In addition, in Grade I patients there are neither obvious neurological manifestations nor spinal degeneration present.

The Grade I patient is usually placed on a limited frequency of visits with the primary goal of correcting any underlying subluxation syndrome that may be observed. Quite often the patient may require daily care for a brief period until significant relief from presenting symptoms is achieved. Remember that in this situation, the subluxation complex may be minimal and, at the same time, chronic.

It is important that the doctor not use the presence or absence of subjective findings to determine whether or not the underlying spinal abnormality has been reduced or corrected. Continued objective findings and proper instrumentation should be considered to ensure that the desired correction of the vertebral subluxation is being attained.

The second phase of managing the Grade I patient usually involves a continued two-to-three-times-per-week assessment of the rate of correction and chiropractic adjustments as indicated. The patient should continue to be monitored until all of the criteria for maximum correction have been attained and the patient is able to perform daily activities without aggravation. Quite frequently, the corrective phase of Grade I patient care is between two to six weeks.

Once it appears that the underlying subluxation has been corrected, it is beneficial to simply monitor the level at which the patient is maintaining their spinal correction, the continued absence of any clinical observations of the components of the vertebral subluxation. During the stabilizing phase of care, the patient should be monitored and adjusted as needed until the spine has become stable and the patient is retaining their correction for extended periods of time. Objective factors may include the restoration of normal function, strength, and flexibility. Sometimes referred to as the "healing phase," the strengthening and stabilizing of the supportive soft tissue structures may take between 6 and 12 weeks in a true Grade I patient.

Grade II

The second classifications of patients you may encounter are those who fall into the Grade II category. The qualifications of this category are that the patient will exhibit a moderate level of pain and frequently reports pain or symptoms in more than one area. The Grade II condition-based patient has symptoms that are worsened or aggravated with activity. At this level, there is no observable spinal deterioration, but often the patient will present with a neurological manifestation. And finally, this patient will often report they have experienced previous episodes or similar problems.

In our practices, we have found that the Grade II patient responds best to daily adjustments when objectively indicated. With effective care directed toward reducing the subluxation complex, the patient usually reports significant relief from presenting symptoms quite rapidly. In fact, with careful spinal analysis and appropriate adjustive techniques, the patient's subjective complaints are usually greatly relieved within the first week or two.

As in all chiropractic care, the elimination of the vertebral subluxation complex is much more important than the temporary relief of the patient's subjective complaints. In Grade II patients, the corrective phase of care is usually significantly longer than in Grade I. We have found that once patients report relief from their presenting complaints, their spines are still structurally flawed and unstable. Great care should be taken to continually discuss the benefits of "spinal correction" with the patient, rather than merely the temporary relief most patients expect. It has been consistently demonstrated in our offices that by continuing to monitor the patient and to work to correct the vertebral subluxation, the patient's spine can be corrected and ongoing condition-based care prevented. For almost 30 years, I have recommended that these patients be checked on a three-times-per week basis, until all of the objective and subjective criteria for maximum correction have been attained, and the patient is able to perform daily activities without aggravation. The correction of this level of patient may average about one and one half to two months.

Just as orthodontists place retainers on their patients after removing braces, so too must we ensure that the patient's corrected, but unstable, spine does not drift back to its original and accustomed, yet subluxated state. Therefore, we always recommend patients reduce their frequency of care in an orderly fashion. Once maximum correction is complete, we begin reducing the patient's level of monitoring to twice a week, then once per week until it has been ascertained that the spine has stabilized and the patient is retaining their correction for extended periods of time with normal function, strength, and flexibility restored. A Grade II patient typically will take 12 to 16 weeks to stabilize once their spine has been corrected.

Grade III

The Grade III patient is the greatest challenge in any chiropractic office. Proper first visit procedures as we have been discussing are mandatory in properly positioning this patient's understanding and expectations of what they should expect in a chiropractic office. Although these patients present in severe pain in one or more different areas, if managed properly, they will become lifelong patients with both respect and acceptance of the doctor and chiropractic.

Not only are these patients in severe and intractable pain when they enter your office, but that pain actually precludes most activities—including employment. Although these patient often have a history of similar complaints and have "been through it before," they are often apprehensive about their ability to "get well this time" and return to work. Thy are worried about their financial survival as much as the current state of their health. With the Grade III patient, your consultation must be in-depth and detailed and your examination a complete and unhurried. The procedures associated with the first day's induction of the patient into your practice will set the stage for their trust and compliance.

You should also be aware and make it understood to the Grade III patient that they may have extensive spinal deterioration or degeneration. This finding alone will be a clue to both doctor and patient that relief, correction, and stabilization will be slow and often not complete. When developing your recommendations with this patient, always strive to advise sufficient time and care to achieve the maximum results possible.

Finally, as in any subluxated patient, they will present with related neurological manifestations. The big difference with the Grade III patient is that these symptoms are usually obvious and extensive. They may range from radiating pain to specific functional insufficiencies. These manifestations are to be thoroughly documented, and quite possibly referral should be considered. In the event of a referral, however, the chiropractic reduction of the causative vertebral subluxation must never be neglected.

The relief care phase of the Grade III patient can be daily-to-multiple adjustments per day, to successfully reduce the vertebral subluxation and the resulting syndrome. Although multiple daily visits may seem excessive to anyone who does not understand what the Grade III patient is experiencing, the patient will gratefully accept those recommendations in the hope of obtaining the desired relief as quickly as possible. This level of care should continue until the patient reports significant relief from presenting symptoms. Under conservative chiropractic care, it has been my experience that the Grade III patient will often respond dramatically and be significantly improved within 10 to 14 days.

As in all levels of patient care, a major component in properly caring for your Grade III patient is to strive to successfully bring the patient past initial intensive relief care, and to effect a level of correction and stability that will return this patient to a healthy, productive lifestyle. Because of the destructive nature of a subluxation complex that has developed to this point, the frequency of corrective care will be similar to Grades I and II (three times per week until maximum correction in attained), but will quite often take a longer period of care to accomplish. Unfortunately, because of the level of spinal deterioration, total correction may be impossible to achieve. Typically, we see the need for 10 to 16 months of care to effect such correction.

As the objective criteria for the correction of the patient's various subluxations are attained, the patient may then be reduced in their frequency of care and monitored for any relapse until the spine has stabilized and the patient is retaining the adjustment for extended periods of time with normal function, strength, and flexibility restored.

Always remember that every patient is different and presents with a unique set of circumstances. The previous description of care for the various levels of patient only provides suggestions and basic guides. While the actual frequency and duration of care will vary, the basic objectives will not. Developing and adhering to a strict one-size-fits-all protocol of care will always cause some patients to receive more care than necessary and others inadequate levels of care. The reevaluation and review process, which we will discuss later, will afford the doctor the ability to make the right decisions in managing their patients. Honesty and integrity are the most important qualities in successful patient management and in building a successful practice.

Step 6-2: Making Appropriate Clinical Recommendations

Concurrent with the triage or grading of the patient, it is helpful to predetermine basic patterns of care (adjustment frequency) into which these patients may initially be placed when making specific recommendations. Predetermined patterns of care, based on the patient's presenting clinical picture, will efficiently and accurately allow the doctor to make objective and clinically proven recommendations for care.

Besides making logical and effective decisions on the patient's clinical status and their initial course of chiropractic care, clinically categorizing the patient and using predetermined objective recommendations based on your clinical objectives will enable you to manage the patient based on specific clinical goals.

Following the decision-making and grading process of the patient, the doctor should then designate the recommended frequency by checking off the appropriate level of recommendations in the case management box on the patient information card. At that point, the CA can develop the appropriate appointment plan. Then, by utilizing the insurance/co-payment worksheet, the CA can also begin to complete the financial arrangements for presentation to the patient following the case report.

During this same time, the CA must have completed transferring a synopsis of the consultation information from the consultation worksheet to the patient information card. The CA also must have assembled all of the case report materials so the case report will go smoothly when the time arrives.

Step 6-3: Building the Relationship— the Case Report

The patient's second visit is equally as important as the initial visit, but for different reasons. On this visit, the patient will enter the office with an entirely new set of concerns. If the first visit went as planned, many of the patient's initial apprehensions will have been dealt with, the patient will have accepted you as his or her doctor, and now be open to the rest of what you have to tell them. This, then, is the next step in building a warm, loving, professional relationship with the patient. This relationship will grow and strengthen with time, and it will potentially be one of the most important relationships this individual will ever form.

By the second visit, the patient now knows that you and your staff are warm and caring individuals, unlike the cold sterile offices of the past. They know you are professional, knowledgeable, and capable. The initial examination was thorough and because of your description of the various tests and their results, they have a good idea of basic findings derived from the examination. And, they know that your fees are reasonable and your policies well planned, well communicated, and patient centered.

However, as the patient returns for the second visit, a totally different set of concerns must be addressed. If these concerns are not adequately dealt with, the establishment of a lifelong doctor-patient relationship will be difficult to develop. At this point, most patients' concerns consist of four basic questions:

1. What is the true underlying cause of my symptoms?
2. What are my options for care?
3. What needs to be done/what can I expect?
4. What can I do to help myself?

The case review now becomes the vehicle for the transmission of the answers for these questions. Properly conceived and delivered, the case review is the single most important tool in helping the patient to understand their situation and the chiropractic approach to helping them. It is also a vital tool in guiding the patient to the proper decision to avail him or herself of the initial three phases of conditioned-based care. It is important to understand that the case review is not a substitute for the patient's ongoing chiropractic education. It is, however, the first step in their basic understanding of what chiropractic is and what you will be doing for them.

As the new patient arrives for the second visit, that person should, as always, be welcomed immediately. They should be addressed by name, shown where to sign in, and then offered a seat:

CA: "Hello, Mrs. Jones. We are all ready for you today. If you will sign in and have a seat, it will just be a few minutes."

It is always helpful for the patient's spouse to come along. Not only does the spouse then understand what their husband or wife is going through, but they also understand the rationale behind your "objective-based" recommendations and will ultimately become a valued ally, rather than a detractor who simply doesn't comprehend chiropractic and the specific objectives of your recommendations and subsequent care.

Whenever a spouse accompanies the patient, everyone in the office, especially the front desk CA, should acknowledge the spouse and make him or her feel as welcome, as comfortable, and as "at home" as possible:

CA: "Is this your husband, Mrs. Jones?

"Mr. Jones, my name is Carol. We're really glad that you came along."

When it is time to take the new patient back to the consultation room, the CA should go into the reception room, call the patient by name, and ask them to follow:

CA: "Mrs. Jones, I can take you back now. Would you and Mr. Jones like to follow me?"

The CA should lead the patient down the hall and into the consultation room. Upon entering the consultation room, the CA should motion for the patient to sit in the proper chair. If the spouse is accompanying, he or she also should be directed where to sit. This prevents the patient (or spouse) from inadvertently sitting in the chair to be used by the doctor and the resulting embarrassment of the doctor having to ask the patient or spouse to move.

The Case Report

The case review is a vital step in the patient education process. It is a time to answer the patient's questions and make honest, straightforward recommendations. It is not a time to "sell" or "close the deal." If the first visit consultation and chiropractic examination were performed properly, the patient should already have great confidence in you and have already decided that they will follow your recommendations. Therefore, if the patient's report is well conceived and presented with compassion and integrity, patient compliance will naturally follow.

The case report is just that, a report of all of the objectives and subjective findings, plus the clinical recommendations for the successful management of the case. It must be delivered in such a way that you inform the patient of the true nature of the cause of their concern. In addition, it is the time to present a plan of action that is comprehensible and logical to the patient and spouse, one that advances the concepts of relief, correction, and future prevention of the problem.

I recommend that a detailed report should always be given to the new patient prior to the initiation of any actual care. If done properly, the case review should be presented in such a way that the patient has all of their questions answered, and completely understands those answers. The patient should leave the consultation room with the attitude of "Wow. That was simple enough. I can't wait to get started."

When you enter the case report or consultation room, you must present a serious, yet friendly aura. Of course you must greet the patient and the spouse, in a sincere manner, and thank the spouse for coming along. To enhance the patients ability to comprehend and learn, the case review should be accompanied by written materials that are easily personalized and that the patient may take home, study, and show to interested friends and relatives. Most importantly, giving both an oral and a written report to the patient serves to reinforce the information by using multiple sensory pathways.

This information should be developed in such a way that it enables the patient to become aware of their problems and understand the necessity of the care that will be recommended. Properly presented, such information should motivate the patient to accept and follow through with your recommendations. When done correctly, the case review will also set up the CA's portion of the second visit, making his or her job of developing the patient's case management plan and attending to financial arrangements appear both logical and straightforward.

The Case Review: Answering the Patient's Four Prime Questions

The actual script of your case review should be one that answers the four basic questions every patient needs to have answered prior to initiating care in your practice. These four important questions are:

1. What is the true underlying cause of my symptoms?
2. What are my options for care?
3. What needs to be done/what can I expect?
4. What can I do to help myself?

If these patient concerns are addressed in an open, honest, and up-front manner, the patient will understand their particular situation, the chiropractic approach to their case, and how their doctor—you—will care for them.

If your case review satisfactorily answers these questions, the patient will understand both the vertebral subluxation complex, its effects, and the processes of properly correcting it. With such understanding will come the desire of the patient to avail himself of the benefits of living subluxation-free. In addition, such an understanding will ultimately lead the patient to make the correct decisions pertaining to following your recommendations and eventually the insight to choose a chiropractic lifestyle for his friends and family.

The first question *(What is the true underlying cause of my symptoms?)* is the primary question that all patients will have on their minds when they enter your office. It must be answered immediately and thoroughly in a manner that your patient will completely understand, and in a way that she will be able to relate it to other individuals in her life.

Most (if not each) of the five components of the vertebral subluxation complex can be revealed to the patient during the initial new patient examination process. Discussing and correlating the patient's case history, their initial chiropractic examination, and the analysis of their x-rays will introduce the concepts of vertebral malposition and spinal distortion, and provide early insights into the concept of nerve impingement as the underlying cause of the patient's major problems.

If your examination and x-rays indicate the existence of any of the five components of the vertebral subluxation complex, each of these should be discussed as they relate to the acuteness and chronicity of the case and its impact on future care and outcomes. Using a check-off list of the five components in your written review will effectively cement these concepts into the patient's consciousness.

Once your patients understand their situation, many may start considering (in the back of their minds) what other modes of care may be available for such a dilemma *(What are my options for care?)*. Addressing such a natural concern in a rational up-front manner will stop most patients from later second-guessing their decision to choose chiropractic. At the same time, they will be able to reply to well-meaning friends and relatives who may not be familiar with the goals of chiropractic care and question the patient's decisions regarding this approach.

At this point, a brief discussion of the two basic options ("correct the cause" or "treat the symptom") that the patient may consider will crystallize in the patient's mind as awareness of the major difference between the chiropractic approach and other approaches to their situation. To make certain the patient understands and accepts the chiropractic approach to caring for their problems, it is important, at this point, to ask the patient to choose which option they wish to pursue. If they indicate they would like to "correct the cause" rather than "treat the symptom" it is likely that you have successfully repositioned the patient's concept of how to most effectively address their situation. Giving the patient the necessary information to correctly make such a decision will usually foster a firm commitment of follow-through and compliance.

Whether the patient broaches the subject of other approaches of caring for their situation or not, it is always helpful to address the situation head-on. It is especially easy when we understand that, when vertebral subluxations are present (and there is no evidence of other pathology or structural damage), chiropractic is indeed the approach of choice.

Then, with the understanding of the cause of their problem and their options, the patient will naturally want to know how they should proceed in successfully addressing such a dilemma and what they can expect as far as case management and prognosis. *(What needs to be done/*

what can I expect?) At this point, your case review should describe a specific program of care designed to accomplish three specific objectives that are logical and acceptable to the patient.

The objectives to be attained during the initial condition-based phase of care include symptomatic relief, subluxation correction, and spinal stabilization. We have found over the years that by making our recommendations "objective-based," our patients more naturally understand and become committed to their care and to attaining these set objectives. The main benefit of objective-based recommendations is that their attainment can be demonstrated and quantified by established examination and x-ray protocols. Progress in attaining these objectives is the rationale for all decision making for future care, and in communicating such needs to the patient throughout the course of the patient's condition-based phase of care.

Finally, the development of an effective doctor-patient relationship involves the accepting of specific responsibilities by each party. Though the patient has already committed to getting the care they need, providing and discussing specific behaviors and rules that will help the patient help themselves is a good way to wrap up the review and to solicit patient cooperation in all areas of their care. By framing this topic as a patient question *(What can I do to help myself?),* you can easily provide a list of specific suggestions for appropriate patient behaviors that the patient will readily accept. This set of rules (suggestions) may be different for each practitioner, but laying early groundwork will set the stage for your acceptance of the patient and their undertaking of the appropriate activities that will allow them to enjoy the best results possible under chiropractic.

Following the case review, the CA should enter the room and review the financial aspects of the case, and begin to develop the "multiple appointment program" (discussed later) that will provide an effective plan for the clinical management of each case.

Case Review Script

The following review script is an example of the case review that may be utilized with each patient during the second visit. You may use it as an outline for your own case review or memorize and use it as is. The booklet can serve as a template for each review and make the utili-

◆ 7 Solutions for Building Your Proactive Chiropractic Practice ◆

Chiropractic

Case Review
&
Clinical
Recommendations

For:

_____

MEYER CHIROPRACTIC OFFICES

Michael S. Meyer, D.C., F.P.A.C., F.I.C.A

zation of this report easily incorporated into your new patient education program.

Doctor: "Good morning, Mrs. Jones. Today I would like to take a few minutes to review with you what we determined through yesterday's consultation, examination, and x-rays to be the important aspects of your case. Then, I would like to give you an overview of how I will recommend that your case be handled.

"To do this, I have developed a case review booklet that contains all of the items that we need to discuss. As we review your concerns, you'll probably have some questions that will come to mind, but if you hold them until we are done, we will probably answer them for you in their proper sequence."

Introduction: Four Questions

Doctor: "Mrs. Jones... There are four questions that I believe all patients should ask their doctor about any health concern they may have. But, rather than take a chance you might not ask them, I have designed this booklet to give you those answers—even before you ask them."

At this point, you should turn to the case review booklet and open it to the first page revealing the four prime questions that each patient should ask. Before going directly into the case review, it is helpful to break the ice by reviewing each question and explaining it and its importance.

Doctor: "First, I believe that the patient should always have a working knowledge of what their problem truly is. So the first question I am sure is uppermost in your mine is: 'What is the true underlying cause of my symptoms?'

"Next, you should ask: 'What are my options for appropriate and effective care?' I think that a properly informed patient should have knowledge of any other options there might be in approaching this problem. So, I will touch on the basic concepts of other approaches other than chiropractic. Then you can make you own decision as to how you wish to proceed.

THERE ARE FOUR IMPORTANT QUESTIONS EVERY PATIENT SHOULD ASK...

☞ *WHAT IS THE TRUE - UNDERLYING <u>CAUSE</u> OF MY SYMPTOMS?*

☞ *WHAT ARE MY OPTIONS FOR APPROPRIATE CARE?*

☞ *WHAT NEEDS TO BE DONE & WHAT CAN I EXPECT?*

☞ *WHAT CAN I DO TO HELP?*

"Once you understand the cause of your concern and your options for addressing this situation, you will naturally want to know: 'What needs to be done?' or 'What can I expect as far as the type and amount of care and time needed to resolve the situation?'

"And last, I just love it when patients ask me: 'What can I do to help myself?' This indicates a patient who truly wants to get better and wants to cooperate—even play an active role in doing whatever is necessary to get the best results possible. Therefore, we are going to discuss some of the things you can do to help as well.

"Did you have any other questions that I have missed?"

Always make certain these four questions seem logical and obvious to the patient. By asking if the patient has any other questions, you will be further lowering the patient's apprehension level, allowing them to feel actively involved in the review, thereby letting the patient know that you are open and willing to answer all of their questions and address all of their concerns.

Question One: "What is the true underlying cause of my symptoms?"

Doctor: "First, if you'll remember, yesterday we performed a very through orthopedic, neurological, and chiropractic examination. And, you will also remember that several of the tests were abnormal or seemed to increase your complaints. Those tests gave us a lot of insight into the structures that were involved. (Here you will list any involved structures indicated by exam by using check-off boxes on page two of the review booklet.) Basically, the examination revealed that your primary symptoms seemed to be coming from an involvement of the muscles, nerves, and possibly even a disc in your spine.

"So, to get a better idea as to the cause of these involvements, we took a set of x-rays, which gave us a lot more insight into why these structures were involved."

At this time, turn on view boxes illuminating the patient's x-rays. Briefly point out the basic structures exhibited on the views. This will better orient the patient as to what they are viewing. Following the quick overview, you should point out the suspected areas of subluxation and any possible structural and neurological effects of possible subluxations at this level.

> **Doctor:** "Besides the apparent nerve interference, muscle spasm, and disc involvement we found during the examination, your x-rays revealed a loss of normal positioning of a few of the bones in your spine, which may be the underlying cause of all of these other findings." (Demonstrate on films and model spine, and draw the four-vertebra diagram in the booklet.)

The four-vertebra diagram makes the vertebral subluxation simple and logical on the patient's level. With this graphic they can see the anatomical relationships within the spine, and understand the dynamics of several components of the vertebral subluxation complex. I recommend that you use several different colors when drawing in the various spinal structures. This gives the sketch more impact and makes it more understandable. Using colored pencils, Magic Markers, or china markers you can make the bones black, the spinal cord and nerves yellow, the disc green, and the muscles red. Experiment with different colors and types of markers, but most of all, practice this drawing. I have often said this single sketch has been worth millions to my practice in simple patient understanding.

Nerve Impingement

As you draw in the spinal cord and the spinal nerves, the following dialog will begin to introduce the patient to the chiropractic concept of nerve impingement and its effect on the patient's physical functioning. The understanding of this one simple concept is critical for the patient to have a working understanding of the chiropractic principle and their ensuing care in your office.

> **Doctor:** "When this misalignment occurs, these bones often impinge upon the spinal nerves and disrupt the nerve signals between the brain and the body. This interference causes pain, but most importantly, it may disrupt and cause malfunction in the areas targeted and controlled by these nerves. (Safety pin cycle)
>
> "This disruption of the nerve messages then leads to the pain and symptoms of ill health that brought you to our office."

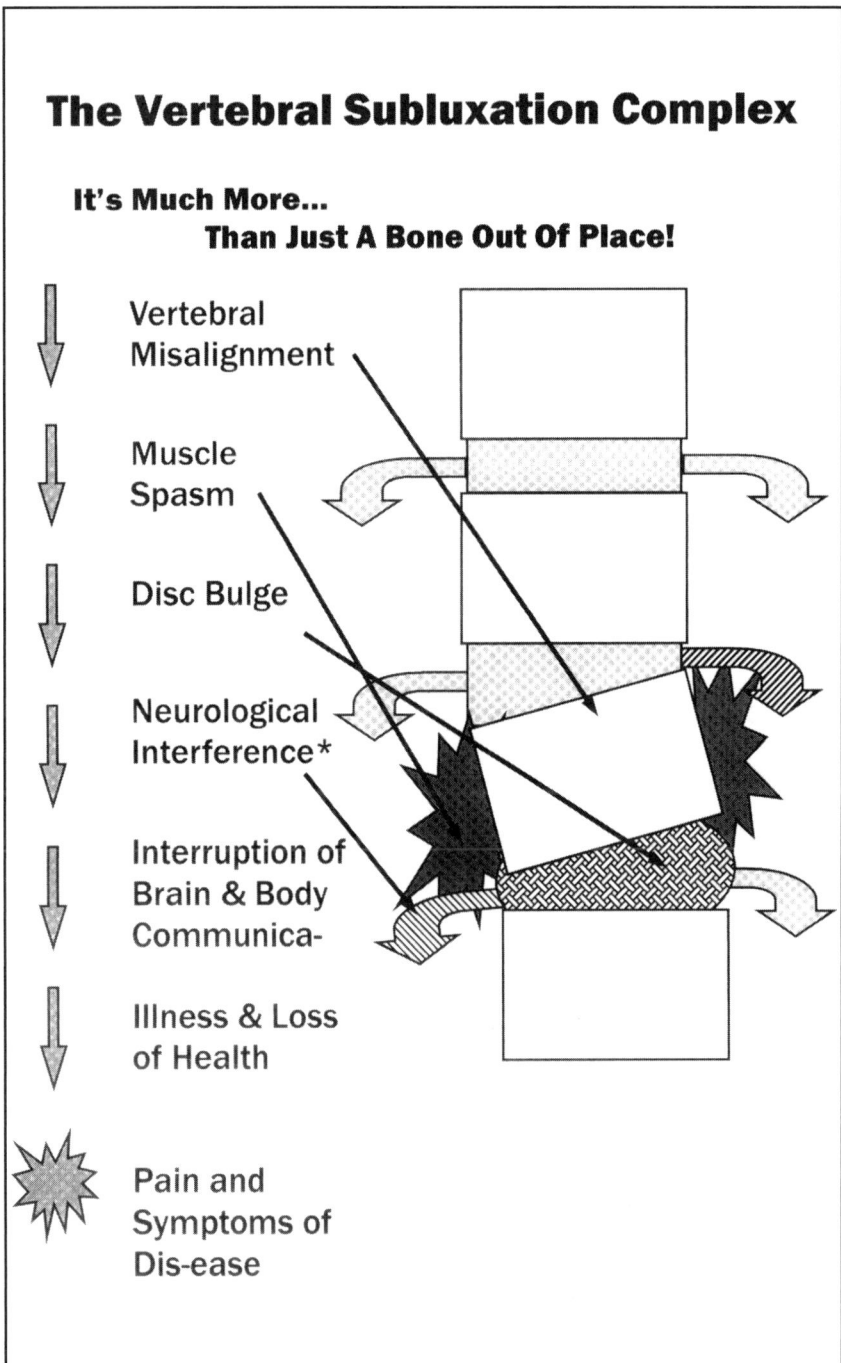

Four Vertebra Diagram

Disc Involvement

Many patients who will initially enter your office with back pain are sometimes concerned that their problem may be a "slipped disc." Those more knowledgeable may wonder if they have a "herniated disc." I have found that a simple explanation of the dynamics and actions of the inter-vertebral disc will set the patient's mind at ease, and help them to better understand the mechanism of the subluxation complex—especially as it relates to the disc.

> **Doctor:** "At the same time, this misalignment (which is called a vertebral 'subluxation') also produces an abnormal pressure on the inter-vertebral discs and may produce disc problems such as bulging, herniation, or over the long term, degeneration of the disc and spine. In your case, the tipping of the vertebra is producing some pressure, possibly forcing some bulging. The test we performed yesterday did not indicate a herniated or ruptured disc. (If true.)
>
> "However, we are concerned with the apparent pressure being exerted on the structure, and we will work to normalize that as quickly as possible."

Muscle Splinting (Spasm)

By discussing the actions of the paravertebral musculature in its attempt to splint and stabilize the spine, you can make a good case as to why muscle-relaxing drugs may set the patient up for further injury. Here also is a good time to demonstrate to the patient the body's wisdom and ability to maintain and even protect itself, while discussing the potential benefits of symptomatology.

> **Doctor:** "Often, to reduce the harmful effects of the vertebral subluxation, the body tries to protect and correct itself by contracting and splinting the surrounding muscles (just like putting a cast on a broken bone), thus limiting movement and creating warning signals we interpret as pain. As you can see, this is a protective mechanism your body uses to prevent more severe and possible permanent damage to the other structures of the spine. This explains the muscle spasms that we have found."

Discussion of Altered Nerve Transmission and the Patient's Health

Now that the patient has a good feel for the actual mechanics of the vertebral subluxation and the structures involved, the chiropractic principle and the safety pin cycle should be introduced. You need to only touch on this subject, since you will be conducting ongoing discussions with the patient throughout the ensuing weeks of care.

Doctor: "In the end, we have arrived at a clinical conclusion of a problem that is scientifically termed a vertebral subluxation complex.

"As you can see, the vertebral subluxation complex is much more than a 'bone out of place.' The danger of such a condition is the misaligned vertebra may impinge upon the spinal cord and nerves. When this occurs, it may alter the transmission of the nerve impulses (messages) between the brain and the body.

"This impingement disrupts the overall coordination of the body and the normal function of cells, tissues, and organs. It often produces pain and eventually structural degeneration.

> ### *The Vertebral Subluxation . . .*
> - Impinges on the spinal cord and nerves.
> - Altering the transmission of nerve impulses (messages) throughout the nervous system.
> - Disrupting the normal function of cells, tissues and organs.
> - Leading to dysfunction, inability to adapt, & eventually sickness & dis-ease.

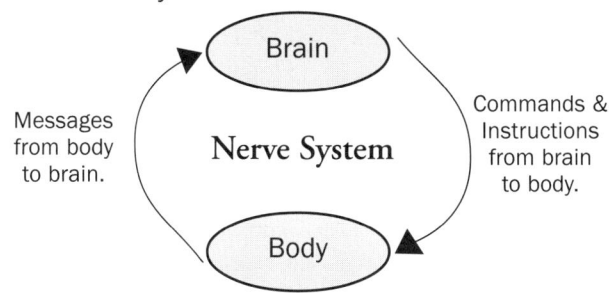

Subluxation Effects

"When this happens, the body's ability to adapt, regulate itself, and function normally is impaired. Ultimately, this impairment causes the body to malfunction, breakdown, and become sickly.

"As you may already be experiencing, the pain and ill-health caused by vertebral subluxations can result in problems in family relationships, the inability to enjoy social activities, diminishment of your capacity to concentrate and to think rationally, plus it threatens your ability to work and possibly your financial survival.

"In this light, chiropractic's greatest role is not to simply relieve your pain, but to correct this challenge to your health and restore your body's ability to adapt, regulate itself, and function in a healthy way. Do you agree?

"Knowing this, Mrs. Jones, your next logical question is..."

Question Two: "What are my options for caring for a health challenge like this?"

Doctor: "Basically you have two options to choose from in addressing this situation. First, there is the approach that attempts to 'treat the symptoms' by using such common means as painkilling drugs to mask and hide the pain, or muscle relaxants that paralyze the muscles that are trying to support your spine to prevent any further damage. Sometimes patients choose surgery that removes the vital disc material or severs nerves to stop the pain. Or, they may even opt for only a few adjustments to temporarily give some relief. In many instances, patients and their doctors prefer to do nothing at all and just learn to live with their situation!

"On the other hand, the chiropractic approach is to work to correct the cause of your troubles by improving the vertebral position, restoring more normal spinal function, reducing the impingement on the nervous system, and restoring function, adaptation, and health.

"So at this point, Mrs. Jones, the decision is up to you. How would you like to proceed with your care? Are you interested in attaining merely temporary relief...or should we proceed with care directed toward correcting and strengthening your spine and ultimately enhancing your overall health for the long term?

"The next question is..."

Patient Options for Care

To care for each patient both ethically and with honesty, the doctor must give the patient all of the information needed to make an informed decision as to how they may proceed with their care. It is the patient, however, who must make the final decision on the course of action.

The choices are clear. Does the patient want to merely obtain temporary, symptomatic relief, or to embark upon a path designed to correct the real—underlying cause of their health concerns. THE VERTEBRAL SUBLUXATION.

Option "1"

The most common approach by many doctors is to merely TREAT THE SYMPTOMS, without correcting the underlying cause. This may be attempted by:
- Pain killing drugs to mask the pain.
- Muscle relaxants to paralyze muscles.
- Drugs to inhibit or stimulate function.
- Surgical intervention.
- Physical therapy to treat the involved tissues.
- Just a few adjustments to provide temporary relief of the pain.

Option "2"

The recommended approach is to strive to CORRECT THE CAUSE—the Vertebral Subluxation.

By utilizing a gentle and safe procedure known as a "Chiropractic Adjustment," the Vertebral Subluxation and it's components may be reduced, corrected, and eventually stabilized by working to:
- Improve the vertebral position.
- Stabilize the spine.
- Reduce nerve impingement.
- Normalize communication & control between the brain and body.
- Restore function, adaptation, health normal and wellness.

Options for Care

Question Three: "What needs to be done to begin to successfully address both your immediate concerns and your long-term interests?"

Three Objectives of Chiropractic Care

Every patient is different, yet there are three specific objectives that are appropriate for all cases:

OBJECTIVE ONE — CRISIS / RELIEF

The initial phase of care must be directed toward gaining control of the presenting complaints by:
- Correcting the vertebral misalignment.
- Decreasing the neurological impingement.
- Alleviating the pain and other symptoms.

MANAGEMENT: _____

ESTIMATE: _____ days/weeks.

OBJECTIVE TWO — CORRECTION

Maximum stabilization is essential for long-term success and the return of health. During this phase, our efforts will be directed toward:
- Health of the muscles & support tissue.
- Stabilization of neurological function.
- Long-term restoration of spinal stability.
- Normalization of function & health.

MANAGEMENT: _____

ESTIMATE: _____ days/weeks.

OBJECTIVE THREE — STABILIZATION

Continued monitoring & prevention of the subluxation complex with special attention given to maintaining spinal integrity & monitoring for stability and long-term correction.
- Secure normal neurological function.
- Long-term restoration of spinal stability.
- Normalization of function & ability to adapt.
- Body working at optimal state of health.

MANAGEMENT: _____

ESTIMATE: _____ days/weeks.

PLEASE NOTE: The above is an estimate based upon the known circumstances of your case. The actual care needed will be determined as the above objectives are achieved.

Doctor: "While we know that every patient is different, there are still three major objectives we need to reach in order to obtain the goals we just spoke of. First, we want to afford you as much symptomatic relief as quickly as possible. To get to that point, we are going to work with you on a daily basis until you report that you are feeling better. Given everything we know about your case, I estimate that within several days you will be noticing major improvements in your symptom complex.

"Once your symptoms are under control and you are more comfortable, we will begin the process of actually correcting the underlying vertebral subluxation complex and restoring normal spinal and neurological function. During this phase, you will have very few, if any, symptoms. Therefore, we will check you two to three times per week for approximately eight weeks and continue to work to correct and strengthen your spine. During this time, we will be regularly performing the same set of tests that we did yesterday. That way we will be able to actually measure your progress. If necessary, we will then adjust your frequency—even your care—as your evaluations indicate.

"Then, once we have made as much correction as possible, we will monitor your spine on a weekly basis for the next twelve weeks. This will ensure that the supporting structures of the spine have stabilized and that you will maintain your spinal correction on a long-term basis."

(*Note:* The above recommendations are only used for descriptive purposes. Your actual recommendations will, of course, vary with each patient and their particular circumstances.)

Doctor: "Now, Mrs. Jones, does that make sense to you? Do you understand what we are trying to accomplish? Do you see anything that might be a problem in your following through with what needs to be done?"

These last three questions are important and should be asked with a high degree of significance. If there is something that the patient does not understand, or if any portion of the review does not make sense, now is the time to back up and make certain all questions have been answered, that they makes sense, and that the patient has no obstacles to receiving the needed care.

Question Four: "What can I do to help myself?"

Home Care & Special

To give yourself the best chance to enjoy the best results possible, please read and follow these suggestions:

1. Try to get some moderate exercise everyday, but avoid jarring activities. Movement is essential to regain normal muscle tone.

2. It is important that you relax before each adjustment. Try to schedule your visits at a time when you can arrive early and relax for a few minutes before seeing the doctor.

3. Try to avoid any type of strenuous activity for at least three hours after your adjustment. This will help your adjustments hold longer and be more beneficial.

4. Do not miss your appointments or change your adjustment schedule. This could slow the progress in correcting your subluxation and restoring strength and stability to your spine.

5. While you are under active care in our office, <u>do not</u> allow anyone to massage, stretch, or manipulate your neck or spine. Such activities may delay healing and be very dangerous.

6. Avoid extreme bending of your spine in any direction, especially following an adjustment.

7. Set aside some time each day for both mental and physical relaxation. During the initial "relief" and "stabilization" phases of care, try to get at least eight hours of sleep each night.

Other: (list here any additional patient recommendations)
_____
_____
_____

What Can I Do?

Doctor: "Good, now there are several things you can do to help us to be as successful as possible in your care. To give yourself the greatest chance to enjoy maximum results, there are six major suggestions that you need to follow. First... (Review a few of your basic suggestions you want your patients to follow.)

"Do you have any concerns that you may not be able to follow these guidelines?"

(*Note:* This is the patient's last chance to voice any concerns or ask any questions during this review. Do not rush. Instead, hesitate long enough for the patient to formulate a response.)

Introduce Financial Review and Multiple Appointment Program

Doctor: "Okay Mrs. Jones, if you have no further questions...before we get started on your first adjustment, Carol is going to review with you your insurance and make whatever financial arrangements are necessary. In addition, she will begin to set your schedule of visits for this week. So, if you can tell her what time of day will be most convenient for you she will try to reserve those time for you in advance. When she is done, she will take you to an adjusting room and we will get you started down the path to getting better.

"I will see you in a few minutes..."

Now, as you (the doctor) leave the conference room, the appropriate staff member should simultaneously enter.

Conclusion and Transition to Financial Review

Before initiating any care for the patient, it is necessary that the financial arrangements are understood and agreed upon and that the planning of the patent's schedule of care is completed. The CA should perform both of these functions after the doctor leaves the room.

To ensure a smooth flow, the CA must be near the conference room door, ready to enter as the doctor leaves. The CA's attitude here is as important as any other point of patient contact up to this point. The financial consultation and setting of future appointments should be extremely low stress for both the patient and the CA. If the doctor has done his or her job in preparing the patient for their care, and the CA has properly planned for the financial administration of the patient's account, the financial review will go quickly. Most importantly, the doctor must have presented the patient's case in a logical, understandable manner and obtained the patient's decision as to the type of care desired; plus a commitment to follow through. If the CA encounters any questions or resistance, he or she should have the doctor come back into the consultation room to deal with any matters that were not fully understood by the patient.

Step 6-4: Making Compliance Easy— the Financial Review and Appointment Arrangements

As soon as the doctor has completed the case report and feels comfortable that the patient understands the vertebral subluxation concept and the objectives for correcting its associated components, the CA will review the patient's financial options, make the appropriate arrangements for payment, then set a schedule of appointments.

The Modified Cash Procedure

The following description of payment determination is called the modified cash procedure. It is designed to take all factors of clinical recommendations, time involved, and the patient's insurance coverage into consideration. Followed exactly as presented and presented properly, this procedure will allow the insured patient to utilize all of their benefits—while paying their portion of the incurred costs over the time frame of their initial condition-based care. Besides making the initial few months' out-of-pocket expenses extraordinarily reasonable, this procedure allows the patient to make an investment in their own healthcare, giving them ownership and thereby a sense of involvement and responsibility. It teaches the patient to pay from the beginning, and ultimately sets the stage for the conversion of the patient from initial condition-based care to lifelong health and wellness.

Determining Payments for Major Medical Coverage

Making specific arrangements that are both simple and equitable will allow the patient to obtain needed care, and to pay their deductible and co-pay amounts over the recommended period of initial condition-based care. Handled in this manner, you can remove one of the biggest hurdles that prevent patients from carrying through with their schedule of recommended care. Of course, the CA cannot determine the actual number of weekly payments the patient will make until the doctor completes the recommendations portion of the patient information card and returns it with the recommended level of care noted.

Once the doctor has supplied the appropriate recommendations, the CA then simply plugs in the proper numbers in the insurance/co-payment worksheet according to the recommended level of care. This worksheet is most effective for determining payments for patients with major medical coverage. It accurately factors in the patient's first visit charges, the total costs of the condition-based phase of care, the level of coinsurance, and the patient's deductible amount.

Utilizing this worksheet, the CA can calculate the total costs (to the patient) of the entire phase of condition-based care. He or she can establish the actual weekly payments necessary to satisfy all of the various contingencies. Use of the worksheet is only for the CA and should not be reviewed with the patient since it may confuse the process and make the presentation procedure more complicated than necessary. After the arrangements are completed, the worksheet should be filed and kept in the patient's file for future reference if necessary.

In virtually every case, by using this procedure the amount the patient will be required to pay on a weekly basis will be so low the patient will never question the amount requested. If the amount is questioned, the CA can simply respond that the amount was determined using a formula that factors in the costs of all the recommended care, and the patient's insurance coverage.

> *Note:* The formula should be followed exactly as it appears on the worksheet, regardless of whether the patient's deductible has been met or not.

The financial review for the major medical patient should be an easy task (provided the doctor has delivered a good report and the patient understands and has accepted every aspect of the case

Insurance / Co-payment
(CA/DR Worksheet)

Patient: _____   Date: _____

CASE RECOMMENDATIONS
COMPLETED BY DOCTOR

1st Week: _____

1st Month (_____-_____-_____-_____) ☐ Re-Evaluation ☐ Re-X-Ray
2nd Month (_____-_____-_____-_____) ☐ Re-Evaluation ☐ Re-X-Ray
3rd Month (_____-_____-_____-_____) ☐ Re-Evaluation ☐ Re-X-Ray

Total Recommended Adjustments   _____
Total Recommended Re-Evaluations   _____
Total Recommended Re-X-Rays   _____

CASE FEES
COMPLETED BY CA

1ST VISIT FEES. . . . . $ _____
OFFICE VISIT FEES. . . . . $ _____
RE-EVALUATION FEES. . . . . $ _____
RE-X-RAY FEES. . . . . $ _____

TOTAL CASE FEES. . . . . $ _____

WEEKLY PAYMENT CALCULATOR

$ _____   - $ _____ . . . . = $ _____
  Total Case   Deductible   (a)

$ _____   x 20% . . . . = $ _____
  (a)   (b)

$ _____   + $ _____ . . . . = $ _____
  (b)   Deductible   (c)

$ _____   / 12 WEEKS . . . . = $ _____
  (c)   Weekly Payment

Sample Form: **Insurance Co-Payment Worksheet**

review—especially the objectives of care and the amount of care recommended). This is because the amount of weekly payments as calculated by the insurance/co-payment worksheet will seem almost ridiculously low to the patient.

> *CA:* "Mrs. Jones, I confirmed your insurance coverage yesterday with your insurance company, and they will cover most, but not all, of your care in our office. Based on your coverage, and what the doctor has recommended, I have averaged the cost to you over the next (insert number) weeks. If you pay $ (insert number) at the end of each week, then by the time the initial condition-based phase of your care is completed, your portion should be all caught up.
>
> "Do you have any problems with this amount? If not, would you like to pay it on your last visit of each week?
>
> "Good, if you will look over this agreement, the assignment form, and sign them...we can get started..."
>
> Note: The effectiveness of the CA in designing and presenting the fee and payment policies and procedures is completely dependent on the relationship that has been developed between the CA and the new patient. Most critical, however, is the doctor's ability to perform a thorough consultation and examination, then to present an effective case review with strong, objective-based recommendations and to form a similarly strong relationship with the patient.

Determining Payments for the Cash Patient

The cash patient may present in one of three variations:
1. The patient who has *no* major medical insurance coverage.
2. The patient who *has* major medical insurance coverage but does not wish to use it and wishes to self-file or who refuses to assign the benefits of the policy to the doctor.
3. In many practices—the personal injury patient.

Give the Patient Financial Options

Although most offices may expect the cash patient to pay at the time of service, most patients with problems that require extended or costly care may be unable to budget such amounts. To demand payment in full from the patient only serves to disqualify many individuals from the practice and withholding chiropractic care from those truly needing it. Instead, your practice should have a menu of payment options that are available to the cash patient.

It is always best both for the patient and the practice, as well as your reputation, to be willing to arrange for payments that will allow the patient to receive care without creating a financial hardship for the patient and their family. On the other hand, making up different financial arrangements for each individual patient is surely a recipe for disaster. If financial arrangements are to be made, preset policies are an absolute necessity for the CA to function effectively in this position. Along with appropriate policies, actual scripts must be developed for effective collection procedures, to reduce stress, and to get the wanted results.

The proper procedures for making financial arrangements with cash patients consist of the following:

1. Conduct a frank, private discussion with every patient as to the anticipated cost of care.

Patients have a right and need to know what they are committing to as they embark on a course of care in your office. At no time should the staff be leery of entering into a discussion concerning fees. If this becomes a problem with your staff, the cause may be a CA who has emotional difficulty dealing with money issues. Usually these hang-ups are deep-seated, stemming from childhood and family influences regarding money. In such cases, this is not the person you want making of financial arrangements with your patients. Replace him or her at once.

Another problem may be that the CA feels your fees are too high and is therefore uncomfortable with their presentation. Unfortunately, they will seldom tell you this. If you feel this may be the case, you need to review your fee schedule carefully and even survey other offices in your area. If you find your fees are out of line, you should adjustment them immediately. If they are not, you should discuss this with the CA and make sure he or she knows that your fees are reasonable and in line with similar practices in the community. Another cause of this type of problem may be a CA who is having financial difficulties and subconsciously believes that if he or she cannot afford your care, then others may be in the same situation. The best solution here is to make sure you are paying your CA appropriately.

Finally, a staff person who is uncomfortable presenting and discussing fees may have a limited understanding of chiropractic and the huge benefits to the patient's health, making the costs of care in your office the best bargain in town. Discussing chiropractic and bringing the staff person to a high level of understanding will greatly improve his or her ability to present fees to patients. This is why keeping your staff and their entire families under care is vital to having a healthy supportive staff who understands the values of, and advocates, chiropractic care for entire families.

2. Give each patient an open and up-front presentation of several acceptable methods of payment.

Allowing the patient to make the decision of how they can handle their financial obligations in your office will empower the patient and prevent the dictatorial policies they have come to expect and resent.

Designing and clearly presenting financial and payment options that are acceptable to both the patient and the practice will result in compliance, goodwill, and high percentages of collections, while allowing the patient to receive the care they need.

3. Establish an agreeable date for payment.

Reaching an agreement with the patient as to when specific payments will be made will create a partnership between the CA and the patient, letting both parties know what is expected. Compliance can only be reached if specific expectations are agreed upon in advance. Here, the CA can be quite liberal in the accommodation of the patient's desire to pay on a certain day, as long as such agreements are honored.

4. Discuss briefly with the patient the consequences of failing to keep an agreement.

With any agreement, there must be an understanding of any consequences of failure to fulfill such an agreement. Whether the consequence is the discontinuation of care or merely the frown of the CA, the patient must know there will indeed be a consequence if a payment is missed. A brief, yet serious, touch on this subject will help the patient stay committed to their agreement.

5. Gain a serious commitment from the patient to make uninterrupted payments and to pay off outstanding balances in full should he or she discontinue care prematurely.

Directive For Disbursement
"Assignment of Insurance Benefits"

By this instrument, I authorize, instruct, and order any insurance company obligated by contractual agreement to reimburse me for allowable professional or medical services to make direct payment to:

_____
_____
_____

This payment shall be credited by the provider directly to my account, and I have agreed to pay (in a current manner) the balance of all charges for professional services over and above the insurance payment.

I also authorize the release of any information pertinent to my case to any insurance company, claims adjuster, or attorney involved in this case.

THIS IS A DIRECT ASSIGNMENT OF ALL BENEFITS TO THIS HEALTHCARE PROVIDER.

_____   _____
Signature of Policy Holder   Witness

_____   _____
Signature of Claimant   Date

A PHOTOCOPY OF THIS DOCUMENT SHALL BE AS VALID AS THE ORIGINAL

Sample Form: **Directive for Disbursement**

Second only to the patient's understanding what is expected of them and what they are committing to financially, gaining a verbal and written commitment is necessary for compliance. A straightforward, eye-to-eye commitment will personally lock the patient into performing as they have promised.

If everything has been handled properly to this point, the commitment will come naturally and gladly. And, while obtaining commitment from the patient is usually easy, obtaining the same commitment from the insurance carrier to make payment to your office and not the patient is another matter. It is therefore mandatory that the patient sign a directive instructing the insurance company to make payment directly to your office. Otherwise, the check will be sent to the patient and a delay will occur in obtaining proper payments.

Possible Arrangements for the Cash Patient

The more payment arrangement possibilities your practice can present, the more you will help ensure that every cash patient can afford to receive the necessary care, satisfy their financial obligations, and become lifelong wellness patients. Ample and appropriate payment options will support the impression that the office is reasonable, concerned, and willing to help the patient. The following are just a few of the possible arrangements that can be made with the new patient. These are presented as possibilities, just to get your creative juices flowing. Design some of your own. Make them creative, fair to both parties, and maybe even fun.

- Payment in full at beginning of care for (insert number) percent discount
- Payment in full at beginning of care—no charge for reexams
- Payment in full at the end of each week
- Weekly payment average of total anticipated care
- Credit card authorization to charge balance at the end of the month

Remember that all arrangements should be designed to make it easy for the patient to stay, pay, and get well. Every effort should be made, however, to have the vast majority of the cost of services paid for by the end of the patient's period of initial condition-based care. If, however,

Patient Agreement
Regarding Non-Insurance Payment Option

We are happy to offer you several choices of payment for the program of care you are about to receive in our office. As an alternative to collecting fees at each visit, we have developed these options to streamline your payments and to remove any financial obstacles. Our intent is to make it both convenient and less costly for you to receive the care that you need.

RECOMMENDED CARE: _____ **VISITS**

ANTICIPATED TIME _____ **WEEKS**

ESTIMATED INVESTMENT $ _____

☐ **Payment in full at beginning of care.**
(15% Discount — Save $_____)

☐ **Credit card authorization** (to charge balance of account at end of week.)
(10% Discount - Save $_____)

☐ **Weekly Payment Average Plan:**
____ post-dated checks in the amount of $_____.
(5% Discount—Save $_____)

☐ **Payment in full after each visit.**

PATIENT AGREEMENT

In selecting the above payment option, I agree:

1. To make uninterrupted payments based on the option that I have selected until my account balance reaches zero.

2. That (unless other arrangements are made) no further care shall be rendered should any payment become seven (7) days past due.

3. That if I discontinue care for any reason (other than discharge by doctor) all outstanding balances shall immediately become due and payable.

4. That if I have pre-paid for my care, and if for any reason I must discontinue care, all unused portions of the advance payment will be returned, less any discount applied.

The above options and all costs associated with my care in this office have been thoroughly explained to me. I wish to participation in this plan of payment for the professional services that I will receive.

_____ _____
Signature of Patient or Guardian *Date*

Sample Form: **Patient Agreement/Cash**

the practice has a large degree of wellness carryover at the end of condition-based care, and, in the judgment of the doctor and the CA, the patient is sincere, payments may be stretched out past initial condition-based care and into the first few months of wellness care.

Once a fair, mutually agreed-upon financial arrangement has been made, it is up to the staff to collect the agreed-upon amounts at the agreed-upon time. Failure of the staff to collect from the patient or failure to enforce these arrangements impairs both the patient's ability to get well and the practice's ability to remain solvent.

Memories sometimes fade and misunderstandings of verbal agreements happen—even with the best intentioned patients. Therefore, besides making specific arrangements for the cash patient to receive the care he or she needs, the patient agreement form is an enormously important aspect for creating an contract for care and the payment of fees. The CA should always review each aspect of this agreement. Each is designed to fairly and diplomatically inform the patient that you are compassionate yet serious about the patient's following through with care, and at the same time honoring their commitments.

For the patient's sake, as well as the financial stability of the practice, fees and collections must be handled with flawless skill, forethought, and judgment. It has been my observation that chiropractors in general are often woefully lax in this area of managing their practices. Usually for the right reasons but with the wrong results, we tend to mess up our financial dealing with patients, leaving the doctor and the practice being taken advantage of, or the patient feeling that the doctor and staff are more interested in their collections than the healthcare they render. For all of the following reasons, please reread this section and make certain your financial policies are well designed, well written, and well presented.

1. Documented studies have shown that patients who are in arrears to their doctor, subconsciously have difficulty allowing themselves to experience positive results. ("Why should I pay, (he or she) didn't help me.")
2. Patients who are behind in their payments or owe their doctor money tend to avoid their doctor and do not receive needed care. Therefore, when patient's accounts are mishandled or not serviced properly, their appointments are more likely to be broken or missed.

3. Strange as human nature is, patients who are behind in payments tend (again, subconsciously) to resent their doctor and seldom refer other potential patients (or worse, refer similar patients).
4. When collection proceedings are instituted, the possibilities of malpractice allegations against the doctor increase.

For these reasons, it is important that collections proceed as agreed upon. All arrangements with the patients should be written on the patient's ledger card or noted on the office computer, and collections made as a routine (and important) part of the CA's job. For all of the previous reasons, you must also pay close attention to the collection percentage in the practice. Anytime your collection percentage falls below 90 to 95 percent, serious inspection must be made into your practice's financial and collection policies and the CA's performance in this area.

Step 6-5: Manifesting the Clinical Plan— the "Map" Procedure

The case management plan and the multiple appointment program are the physical manifestations of your clinical plan of action in each patient's individual case. They are the most important tools you will find to help keep your patient on the proper schedule of care and visit frequency. Ultimately, they give the doctor and your staff the ability to monitor and manage the attainment of the objectives of care that have been recommended to, and accepted by, the patient. Implementing the case management plan allows several appointments to be scheduled in advance, and serves many important purposes. Most importantly, it allows the patient to plan all upcoming obligations on their time around their care in your practice. It also helps you and your staff to follow the patient's progress and to schedule reevaluations and upcoming reports on a timely basis. In addition, multiple appointments facilitate the future scheduling of patients, and block-booking of patients, allowing for both practice growth and stability.

The case management plan is so valuable to proper patient management that space on the patient information card should be devoted to executing this process. A box with the most common case management recommendations given to your patients, based on your technique and

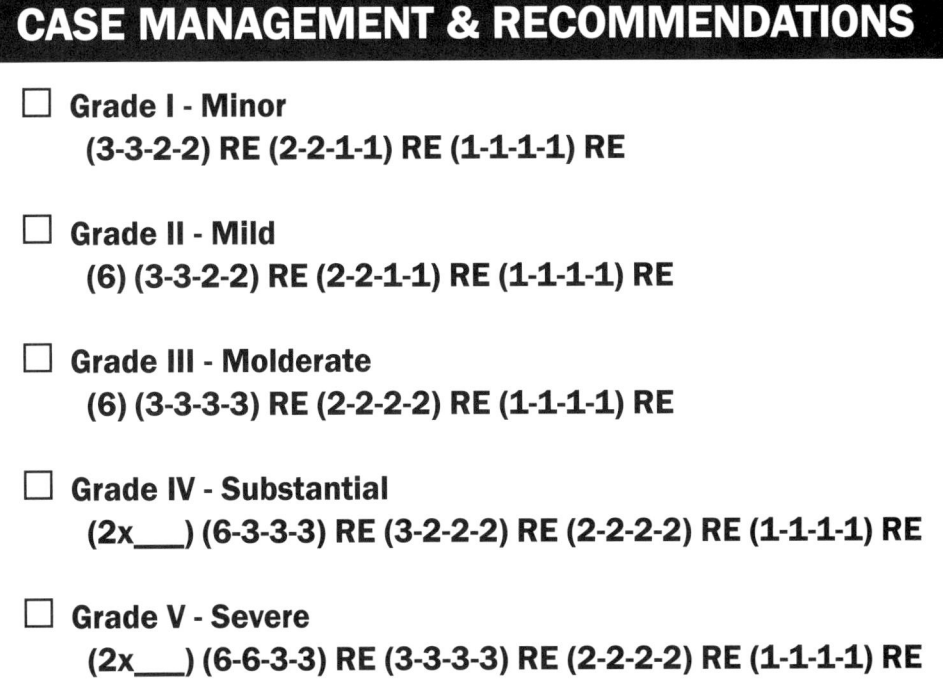

Case Management and Recommendations

anticipated clinical accomplishments, should be included on the patient information card for easy check-off by the doctor and precise communication to the CA. As in the example below, the case management box contains several grades of severity within which patients will present. Following the appropriate first day's procedures, and the grading system associated with making appropriate recommendations, you will easily know to which category the patient belongs, and recommendations can be easily and quickly made.

Also to be included on the patient information card is a generic calendar that will allow the CA to actually record the future schedule of recommended and accepted care for both the doctor and the staff to reference. Having this calendar on the patient information card allows everyone in the practice to see at a glance the progress of the patient throughout the program of initial care. Properly managed, the CA will place slashes ("/") in the appropriate dates as appointments are scheduled and entered into the appointment book. As patients present at

♦ 7 Solutions for Building Your Proactive Chiropractic Practice ♦

RELIEF & CORRECTIVE CARE SCHEDULE

Month	1	2	3	4	5	6	7	8	9	10	11	12	13	14	15	16	17	18	19	20	21	22	23	24	25	26	27	28	29	30	31
Jan																															
Feb																															
Mar																															
Apr																															
May																															
Jun																															
Jul																															
Aug																															
Sep																															
Oct																															
Nov																															
Dec																															

Map Scheduling Calendar

their appointments and progress through their care, the CA then places an opposite slash mark (forming an "X") through that date indicating that the patient kept that appointment. On the next to last scheduled appointment, the CA places an "R" in the box indicating that the patient is to be reevaluated on that visit. On the last visit, the CA should place a "C" in the box indicating to both you and the person scheduling appointments that the patient should be re-consulted with, and the achievements and further objectives of care reinforced on that day.

The Initial Series (First Week)

Many new patients who are in severe pain or ill health will be seen on a daily basis until their symptoms abate or are brought under control.

When the doctor recommends a period of daily visits to the patient, the first group of scheduled appointments should reflect only the first week's schedule and no more. These may be recorded on the patient information card and on an appointment card that has space formatted for several visits (available from most office form catalogs), and given to the patient when completed.

The Second Series

Toward the end of the first week, the same procedure is repeated for the remainder of the following four weeks. Depending on the case recommendations, the CA must remember that a new series of appointments needs to be made for the patient at the end of the first group of appointments. By being prepared and recording the upcoming series on the appropriate dates before the patient's next scheduled visit, the CA can easily and efficiently set up the next series of appointments. Having the dates already written on the appointment card and ready to establish an actual time with the patient, the card may be presented to the patient at the end of the last scheduled visit.

Principally, the second series of visits to be programmed will consist of the patient being seen three or more times per week for the following three to six weeks. We have found it is best to schedule these patients on Monday, Wednesday, and Friday, or Tuesday, Thursday, and Saturday. This strategy spreads their care evenly throughout the week with proper convalescent intervals between visits. Doctors with growing practices who wish to utilize this extremely effective procedure should plan their office hours accordingly. If the doctor does not have office hours on Saturday, then Monday, Wednesday, and Friday, will naturally be the busiest days in the office. Therefore, taking off Wednesdays to play golf would indeed be unproductive and make proper scheduling extremely difficult for patients and staff.

As patients near the end of each series of appointments (especially as they become symptom-free), they will naturally begin thinking of dismissal—or at least reduction of visit frequency. This, however, is easily remedied by scheduling all reevaluations on the *next to the last* appointment, and the ensuing re-report on the last scheduled appointment. This allows you and your staff to procedurally reexamine, re-consult, reinforce, and reappoint the patient when they are most vulnerable to premature dropout.

By having the CA write the initials "MAP" (in red) after the patient's name in the appointment book on the day before the last visit, the CA will automatically be alerted that more appointments must be scheduled. He or she should then check with the doctor following the reevaluation to make sure the patient is on schedule and will continue to be appointed according to the initial recommendations. Then, on the last scheduled visit of the series, the next series of appointments and the appointment card will be ready to be presented to the patient as he or she leaves the office as described previously.

Scheduling Tips—Review

Again, several important points should be considered to properly schedule the patient's multiple visits. These considerations will increase the effectiveness of the patient's care and, at the same time, balance the office's patient load between days of the week.

- ◆ It is the responsibility of the CA at the front desk to administer the multiple appointment program (MAP). It is also their responsibility to report any patient noncompliance to the doctor and to make appropriate notations on the patient information card.

- ◆ As stated earlier, the first step in this procedure begins with the doctor determining what care is necessary for each individual patient and marking it in the proper area of the patient information card. Not only is the doctor's failure to analyze films, complete diagnosis codes, and determine appropriate case recommendations frustrating for he CA, but it is the first step in mishandling the patient and subsequently hampering your ability to properly manage the patient back to health and a better life. Adherence to a methodical procedure for making appointments is crucial. The CA (after the doctor has designated the appropriate adjustment frequency for each patient) should fill out the multiple appointment card with the anticipated *dates* for the first week of care, and then wait to put the actual *times* down after finding out what time is convenient for the patient. This is best done after the case review, at the same time the CA performs the financial portion of the review with the patient.

◆ The CA's script should be short and to the point. The doctor has done the talking for both of them, and the patient understands what the CA is trying to accomplish, so they should have few questions at this point:

CA: "Mrs. Jones, the doctor has indicated that you will be coming in daily for the rest of this week and three times next week. If you could give me an idea as to what would be the best time of day for you to make your appointments, I will reserve those times for you in advance so that we will be certain that the doctor will be available for you at that time.

"Would you prefer mornings or afternoons? Early or late? 10:00 or 11:00? Next week—will Monday, Wednesday, and Friday work for you?"

◆ At that point, the CA should (in the presence of the patient) make a note of the patient's time preferences on the patient information card. After the CA has completed the financial review with the patient, and discussed a preferred time for the patient's appointment, the CA will escort the patient to the appropriate adjusting room.

While the patient is receiving their first adjustment, the CA can then write the appropriate and preferred time on the multiple appointment card, and draw an arrow through the rest of the dates on the card indicating the same time for all visits. The CA may then enter the patient's name with the appropriate times in the appointment book. This card will be presented to the patient following the first adjustment.

Step 6-6: Make the Patient's First Adjustment Momentous

Placing the patient on the adjusting table for the first time is a momentous event for the patient, and an important threshold in the doctor-patient relationship. At this time, the doctor must describe everything that is happening (especially if the technique requires that any type of a mechanized table is used—Thompson, Cox, etc.). This description should include any special orders for the patient such as: taking glasses or jewelry off, removing shirts or loosening belts, specific head and hand placement, movement restrictions, and many others orders that may be applicable to your technique and preferences. At the same time, the doctor must reassure the patient that there will be no tricks, surprises, or pain. The doctor's voice should be low, calm, and reassuring. It is often beneficial for the doctor to place a hand firmly on the patient's scapular or lumbar area as the table starts down so that they become comfortable with your touch.

Placing the Patient on the Adjusting Table

As the patient and table start down, or as you begin to touch or palpate the subluxated area, the concept of the vertebral subluxation complex and the chiropractic adjustment should be restated.

> **Doctor:** "As I mentioned, your nerve system is being disrupted by this spinal bone right here (palpate level of subluxation) that is slightly misaligned and subluxated. This is what is causing your *symptoms*.
>
> "I am now going to begin the process of moving these bones away from the nerves. When I do, you will hear a slight popping sound as the vertebrae begin to realign. It will not hurt and I will be as gentle as possible. As we do, your altered nerve flow will be restored." (Perform adjustment.)
>
> *Note:* This first adjustment should be as gentle as possible and cause no discomfort to the patient. If an audible is effected by the adjustment, the doctor should once again affirm that this is good, that the adjustment was made, and that the first step in spinal correction has been completed.

Post-Adjustment Release Statement

Doctor: "Okay, Mrs. Jones, we have now begun the process of correcting the cause of your problems and normalizing your nervous system. Let's check it again tomorrow. Together, we will keep adjusting those subluxated spinal segments until we have everything that we talked about today corrected." (Reinforce any special orders for home care.)

"Now, if you will come up front with me, Carol should have you scheduled for tomorrow's visit and you can then go home and rest."

Key Points

- Making appropriate and reasonable recommendations for initial intensive care is important for developing patients who will understand the rationale for care, and will accept your advice.
- Doctors must realize that each patient is different and that giving the same recommendations to every patient, independent of their clinical presentation of individual circumstances, is intellectually dishonest and clinically indefensible.
- The case review is a vital step in the patient education process. It is a time to answer the patient's questions and to make honest, straightforward recommendations. It is not a time to "sell" or "close the deal."
- Before initiating any care for the patient, it is necessary that the financial arrangements are understood and agreed upon, and that planning the patient's schedule of care is completed.
- Making specific financial arrangements that are both simple and equitable will allow the patient to obtain needed care, and to pay their deductible and co-pay amounts over the recommended period of initial condition-based treatment, thus removing one of the biggest hurdles that prevent patients from carrying through with their schedule of recommended care.
- If financial arrangements are to be made, preset policies relating to financial arrangements are an absolute necessity for the CA to function effectively.
- The first adjustment should be as gentle as possible and cause no discomfort to the patient.

Solution

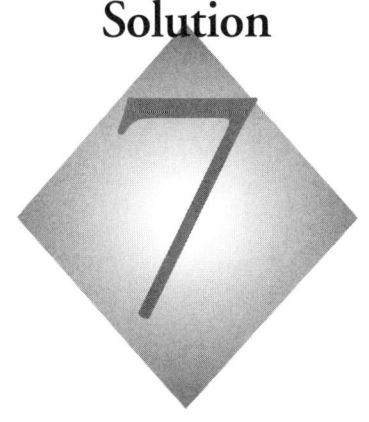

Keep Your Patients Educated, Excited, and Adjusted

Providing the type of leadership that will encourage and excite your patients about the prospect of regained health and a lifetime of wellness is the greatest responsibility of the committed chiropractor. To encourage patients to devote their efforts to getting and staying well, by fulfilling the doctor's clinical recommendations is one of the most important components of being an effective and ethical doctor.

The doctor's untiring emanation of a sense of mission and commitment to the patient and to chiropractic principles draws the patient into the realm of accountability and ownership of their personal responsibility to regain and to maintain their health. Such ownership will lead to compliance, retention, and referrals. The bottom line is that typically it is not the satisfied patient who complies and refers, but the well-educated and excited patient, who is the bedrock of a successful chiropractic practice.

Besides the obvious visceral commitment that must be manifested by the doctor, special procedures, special words, and high standards of patient care are necessary to channel that commitment to the patient.

Such procedures and educational standards should, like the rest of your approach, be a matter of policy and an ingrained component of your established practice procedures.

The following procedures are designed to continue the patient's chiropractic understanding while keeping the patient and doctor abreast of the current status of the patient's progression through the condition-based care phase. These procedures will encourage patient compliance during the most difficult period of patient care. If everything that has been discussed to this point (new patient consultation, examination, case review, objective-based recommendations, financial arrangements, effective chiropractic adjustments, and gaining initial patient commitment) is implemented in your practice, you should now be developing legions of new patients who are well on their way to becoming the ideal patients with whom you will fill your practice.

Step 7-1: Renew the Excitement Before It Fades—the Reevaluation Procedure

Have you ever had a patient who had been coming into your office for several weeks, even months, who appeared to be getting good results, and then suddenly asks, "Doc, how am I doing?" Were you able to honestly and accurately answer the question? Like most doctors, you may have struggled with the answer, sidestepped the question, or brushed the patient off. Not answering this serious question or not addressing the issues behind it is a grave mistake in proper patient management.

But it is a difficult question to answer. The problem is that sometimes patients do not comprehend why they are asking this question, or what they actually need to hear in order to have this question answered satisfactorily. In truth, the patient may be asking a combination of several other questions, such as:

- "Am I still subluxated?"
- "Is chiropractic really helping me?"
- "How much longer do I have to keep coming in?"
- "Why do I still have symptoms?"
- "Is my adjustment holding?"
- " I feel fine. How will you know when my subluxation is corrected?"

Because of the vagueness of such a question, it is often difficult for the doctor to have an honest and satisfactory answer. Moreover, on both an objective and a subjective basis, the day-to-day progress of a chiropractic patient is often incremental and somewhat difficult to measure on each visit.

The patient's objective findings may be better one day and worse the next. They may report feeling relief on one visit and experience exacerbations on the next. Their activity levels will vary from one visit to the next. In short, the day-to-day progress of an average chiropractic case through the relief and correction phase of condition-based care is like watching a child grow. For someone who only sees a particular child every few months, the growth and maturity are much more obvious than for someone who sees that child on a daily basis. The improvements and progress of a chiropractic patient are much like that. Periodic (interval) comparison evaluations will often show tremendous changes that may not have been noted on a daily basis.

Periodic and more detailed evaluations give a much more accurate picture of a patient's progress. Consequently, periodic reevaluations and comparative reviews must be used as the foundation of all ethical patient management procedures.

The reevaluation and comparative report procedures are the most overlooked, yet the most important procedures in the management of a chiropractic patient. Although few doctors actually perform this procedure on a routine basis, those that do have shown greatly improved patient management, compliance, acceptance, and clinical results.

Effective case management is what the reevaluation procedure is all about. The information that such activities provide will help you to determine the clinical results and future case management. At the same time, reevaluation procedures will reinforce to the patient the need for corrective and rehabilitative care. It also affords you and your staff a perfect opportunity to reassess the patient's understanding of the care and the objectives of that care.

Even more importantly, periodic reevaluation simply makes good sense to patients. It provides objective evidence of the effectiveness and necessity of care. It is reinforcement that they have made the right decision in seeking your care. As you explain to patients that these same evaluation procedures that were performed initially will also serve as indicators to determine their progress, they begin to understand the rationale behind your current and future case recommendations, and they begin to get excited about their care all over again. They see their progress. They are reminded where they were and how far the have come. Their commitment to their vision of health, wellness, and the lifestyle it will afford is renewed.

Implementation

Proper introduction of the reevaluation procedure will result in the patient's accepting and appreciating the time spent to update them on their progress. On the day of the reevaluation, the doctor should go into the room with the patient and again explain what will be done and why. Providing a strong rationale will help ensure the patient's enthusiastic acceptance of the reevaluation procedure.

If presented properly, case reevaluation procedures will be reasonable, logical, and well accepted. The patient will easily understand that the goals of their care are based on objective findings and logical conclusions, rather than subjective patient reactions. Implementation of the reevaluation process is a team effort between the doctor and the staff person who is responsible for setting up the patient's multiple appointment programs. The presentation of this procedure actually begins during the initial case review. As the doctor reviews the objective-based recommendations of the case, a point should be made that the attainment of each of these objectives is measurable, and that by using the same tests originally used to determine the patient's problem and the initial need for care, the patients progress can likewise be tracked and analyzed.

For greatest effectiveness, the reevaluation and comparative report should initially be performed every 12 visits on active patients under condition-based care and semiannually on "health and wellness care" patients. Based on your technique, approach, and patient response, x-rays may or may not be taken.

As discussed previously, when setting up the multiple appointment series, the CA should automatically position the reevaluation appointments as recommended by the doctor, being sure to set aside enough time for the reexam to take place on the next to last visit of each series or each three to four weeks.

Consultative Update

Before the clinical portion of the reevaluation is performed, an in-depth subjective consultation update is completed. The doctor (or designated staff person) will question the patient on each initial subjective complaint recorded on the entrance consultation. An important objective of this questioning is to quantify the patient's degree of improvement. An effective way is to simply ask the patient to report progress in percentages (e.g., headaches are 80 percent better, allergies 50 percent better, etc.), and/or in terms of frequency (e.g., headaches are only once a week instead of daily, etc.). Another effective means to evaluate the patient's subjective reports is to use a visual analog scale that renders a numerical value to their complaints during the initial consultation and at the time of reevaluation. The progressive evaluation on the following page offers the benefits of each of these means of evaluating the patient's progress.

Prior to the patient's visit, the CA should transfer the primary entrance complaints onto the progressive evaluation form from the initial consultation. The patient will again be placed in the initial conference area where the doctor will review and ask the *patient* to mark the level of improvement in each area. The doctor will then complete (in a consultative manner) each of the other items on the form.

> **Doctor:** "Mrs. Jones, today we are going to perform the same tests we did on your first visit. This way we can measure your progress to this point.
>
> "First, let's talk about how you have been feeling recently—compared to when we first started.
>
> "Initially, you were concerned about (describe initial complaints). Compared to where we started, can you mark on this scale (progressive evaluation form—side one) where you feel you have progressed to today?"

Continue with each original complaint until all have been discussed and the degree of subjective improvement is quantified.

Progressive Evaluation & Patient Update

Patient: _____ Date: _____

- Check the level of improvement in your symptoms since you began care:

  a. _____ ☐ No Change ☐ ☐ ☐ ☐ ☐ ☐ ☐ ☐ ☐ Symptom Eliminated
  b. _____ ☐ No Change ☐ ☐ ☐ ☐ ☐ ☐ ☐ ☐ ☐ Symptom Eliminated
  c. _____ ☐ No Change ☐ ☐ ☐ ☐ ☐ ☐ ☐ ☐ ☐ Symptom Eliminated

- In what ways has your lifestyle changed since beginning care in our office? _____

- Are there any activities that you are still unable to perform? _____

- How would you describe your health now, as opposed to when chiropractic care was initiated in this office?

  Overall sense of well-being: ☐ No Change ☐ ☐ ☐ ☐ ☐ ☐ ☐ ☐ ☐ Symptom Eliminated
  Energy levels: ☐ No Change ☐ ☐ ☐ ☐ ☐ ☐ ☐ ☐ ☐ Symptom Eliminated
  Soundness of sleep: ☐ No Change ☐ ☐ ☐ ☐ ☐ ☐ ☐ ☐ ☐ Symptom Eliminated
  Overall quality of life: ☐ No Change ☐ ☐ ☐ ☐ ☐ ☐ ☐ ☐ ☐ Symptom Eliminated

- Additional Comments: _____

Sample Form: **Progress Evaluation (consultation)**

◆ Keep Your Patients Educated, Excited, and Adjusted ◆

PROGRESSIVE EXAMINATION

POSTURE & MOVEMENT

Postural Analysis

Head Tilt	☐ Lt	☐ Rt	+ ___
Shoulder Tilt	☐ Lt	☐ Rt	+ ___
Pelvic Tilt	☐ Lt	☐ Rt	+ ___

Weight Bearing

Weight: ___
Distr: ☐ Lt ☐ Rt + ___
Stability: ___

Lumbar Ranges of Motion

	Degrees	Pain
Flexion	___ /90	___
Extension	___ /45	___
L. Rot.	___ /30	___
R. Rot.	___ /30	___
L. Flex.	___ /30	___
R. Flex.	___ /30	___

Cervical Range of Motion

	Degrees	Pain
Flexion	___ /45	___
Extension	___ /45	___
L. Rot.	___ /80	___
R. Rot.	___ /80	___
L. Flex.	___ /45	___
R. Flex.	___ /45	___

NERVE SYSTEM

Reflexes

	Lt.	Rt.
Biceps	___	___
Triceps	___	___
Extensors	___	___
Patellar	___	___
Achilles	___	___

Neuro-Ortho Testing

For Comp: ___
Max Comp: ___
Sh Dep: ___
Distract: ___
Valsalva: ___
Cranial Nerves: ___
Dermatomes: ___
Toe Walk: ___
Heel Walk: ___
Rhomberg: ___

Observation / Notes / Other:

MUSCLE & STRENGTH

Circumference

	Lt.	Rt.
Thigh	___	___
Calve	___	___
Biceps	___	___
Forearm	___	___

Neuro-Ortho Testing

SotoHall: ___
S.L.R: ___
Braggard: ___
Leg Drop: ___

Dynamometer

Lt Hand ___
Rt Hand ___

Vitals

Blood Pressure:
Lt ___ / ___
Rt ___ / ___

VBA: ___
Subclavian: ___
Carotid: ___
Heart: ___

PALAPATORY EXAMINATION

MS	TP	SP	TP	MS
		OC		
		C1		
		C2		
		C3		
		C4		
		C5		
		C6		
		C7		
		T1		
		T2		
		T3		
		T4		
		T5		
		T6		
		T7		
		T8		
		T9		
		T10		
		T11		
		T12		
		L1		
		L2		
		L3		
		L4		
		L5		

Sacrum

Sample Form: **Progress Evaluation (examination)**

The Reexamination

After the re-consultation, you should proceed to re-perform all chiropractic, orthopedic, and neurological tests that were originally positive. In addition, always measure each and every range of motion (cervical and lumbar) and reevaluate the patient posturally, circumferentially, and weight-bearing. Just as in the initial exam, the reexam should be a "talking" exam where you will explain what each test demonstrates, as well as how it has changed from when it was originally performed.

> **Doctor:** "Okay, now let's perform the same tests we did on your first visit, and compare these clinical findings to what we found originally."

At that point, you should move through the entire examination and verbally compare the results of each initial examination procedure with the patient's present status.

> **Doctor:** "Mrs. Jones, this test is called the cervical compression test—it indicates nerve root compression in the neck. Do you remember that this produced significant pain when I first performed it? It appears that we are successfully relieving the nerve impingement that was initially present."

Continue in a similar manner with the rest of the various tests and measurements.

Most enlightening to the patient is for the examiner to note any changes in the patient's postural orientation and the improvements thereto. Such changes are easily seen by the patient and will lead to a high level of acceptance. If the initial examination was performed properly and all positive indications of the various components of the vertebral subluxation complex imprinted in the patient's mind (by both word and pain), the patient will recall the original degree of discomfort presented with each specific procedure. Both consciously and unconsciously, patients will recollect the original subjective and objective problems that brought them under care in the first place.

Once the reexam is complete, you may adjust and dismiss the patient for the day, if indicated.

Doctor: "Mrs. Jones, now that we are done with your progress evaluation, we know there has been significant improvement in your symptomatology. I would like to sit down between now and your next visit and correlate our findings and determine your actual rate of improvement. Let us continue to work on (area of continued concern) today and I will update you on your progress on Friday."

The Comparative Report

When the patient returns for the last scheduled appointment of their current multiple appointment series, the doctor should then review with the patient the results of the comparative exam that was performed on the previous visit. It should be emphasized that the comparative report should be done with seriousness and high intention—that is, both energy and importance should be given to the comparative report. This is one of the most critical components of patient case management.

When you enter the room with the patient, you must look warm and relaxed. Then, sitting next to the patient you may begin the comparative report by explaining the reason for the reevaluation and the hoped-for results. (This may be done in the regular adjusting room.)

Doctor: "Mrs. Jones, before I check you today, I want to review with you the results of your reevaluation last week. We performed this reevaluation so that we can measure precisely how much progress you have made, and to give you an idea of where we need to go from here. First of all, let me review your examination findings..."

Review the original and current subjective findings, comparing the initial consultative information with the most recent. This should be easy to do, by reviewing the reevaluation form that the patient completed on the previous visit. Then, by turning the form over you may tie it all together and confirm the patient's subjective reports with the objective findings from the reevaluation.

In doing so, it is important that the doctor review and ask the patient to remember each positive aspect of the examination. Properly designed, the examination demonstrates the presence or absence of each component of the subluxation complex. Review each one of these and again describe the presenting component as documented on the initial examination. Then, with each improved finding the patient will be more and more satisfied that they have made the right decision to commit to complete the three phases of condition-based care. If the patient is still in one of the three phases of condition-based care, with this level of satisfaction and understanding, they will naturally want to continue on to the next level of care. If they have completed the "relief" portion, "correction" and "stabilization" care is the natural next step. If they have completed stabilization, you will now be able to easily transition them into lifelong wellness-care patients. With the development of more and more of these patients, you will be climbing another step on your stairway to success.

Be aware too that the objective findings may not bear out the subjective reports of improvement by the patient. Again, the patient should be reminded that, just as was explained in the initial case report, the symptoms of the vertebral subluxation complex will often resolve long before the underlying correction has taken place.

Doctor: "To give you an idea as to where you are, Mrs. Jones... you are (right on, ahead of, or behind) schedule. You are (not quite, exactly, progressed ahead of) where I had anticipated you'd be by today.

"At this point, your low back is 75 percent better, your stomach problems are 50 percent, and the numbness in your hands is 30 percent better.

"Again, you are progressing (ahead of, right on, or behind) schedule. At this point, my recommendations are that we...

- Continue as I described in your initial report and reduce your frequency to two visits per week for the next 60 days" (or give further recommendation to patient explaining which phase of care the patient is moving into and the objectives of such care).

- (If patient is ahead of schedule) "... decrease your frequency of care even more than I had initially anticipated. At this point you are actually past the relief phase of your initial intensive care and we are now going to concentrate on correction of the vertebral subluxation."

- (If patient is progressing slower than expected.) "Continue at the same frequency of care that we have been on until we reach the level of improvement that I expect and you want. In addition we will also change our adjusting techniques slightly and start you on a different set of exercises."

"I have asked Carol to set you up for visits per week for the next four weeks. If we continue at this pace, I am hopeful we will have the remaining distortion corrected and ready to concentrate on getting you on a program of strengthening, rehabilitating, and reconstructing your spine at that point. Do you have any questions?"

Note: If the patient has completed the initial three objectives of the condition-based care and all objective findings of the subluxation complex have been significantly resolved, the patient will then be classified as a "wellness patient." At that point, the CA should set them up with a "standing" appointment based on the doctor's further recommendations. As an example, if you recommend that the patient be checked for vertebral subluxations on a biweekly basis, the CA should try to set an appointment routine for the first and third Friday at the same time. (These patients may also appreciate receiving a series of multiple appointments and reserving their special time slot well into the future.)

The patient will also now be converted to a wellness patient with a new payment schedule applying and no insurance reimbursement expected.

Step 7-2: Help Patients Express Their Excitement—Make Wellness a Family Event

At this point in the patient's care, he or she should have a firm understanding of their progress thus far. As well, they should have a growing understanding of real health and true wellness and how chiropractic care fits into this paradigm. They will have formed strong belief systems in the efficacy of chiropractic care. Moreover, a strong relationship of trust and confidence in the doctor will have formed at this point as well. With the further understanding and documentation of such progress (as is generally demonstrated in the reevaluation process) comes renewed enthusiasm and further acceptance. This provides you, the doctor, with an excellent opportunity to delve into the health concerns of the patient's family, better serve the patient and the community as a whole, and begin the process of availing the chiropractic care to any other family members who might also need it.

Besides giving you the important initial information about hereditary possibilities and lifestyle effects, the "family health history form" (see page 276) now becomes an excellent source of information about family members who may have or be developing subluxations and resultant health problems chiropractic can effectively address. By referring to this form at this point in the patient's chiropractic life, you can quickly, sincerely, and effectively explore ways to better serve the rest of your patient's family.

> **Doctor:** "Mrs. Jones, before we check you today, there is one other matter I would like to discuss with you. When you initially filled out the family health history form, I noticed your sister is experiencing similar problems. Have you discussed your case and the results you've enjoyed under chiropractic care with her?"

Allow the patient to respond, and ask all further appropriate questions. The more information the patient will share with you about this family member, the more likely they will come to see the possibilities and wisdom of getting them under chiropractic care. Here, performing a brief new patient consultation—in absentia—may be indicated.

Following the brief information gathering, you should proceed as if this family member lives in another town (unless you know differently). An offer to send information and to recommend a doctor in their area sounds both compassionate and high-minded.

> **Doctor:** "As you can imagine, I am excited with the changes we are seeing in your nervous system. It's very possible your sister could enjoy similar results. If you would like, tell Carol where she lives, I would be happy to help her find a good doctor in her area. Also, I will send her some information about chiropractic."

More often than not, the patient will relate that her family member actually lives in the immediate community. At this point, you can then offer to provide him or her with a complimentary consultation and examination, to see if chiropractic might help.

> **Doctor:** "If she lives here in town, why don't you bring her with you on your next visit and we can see if chiropractic can help her too? I will give you a complimentary consultation and examination card before you leave today."

You can then proceed to adjust the patient. When completed, you should personally escort the patient to the front desk and dismiss the patient with the referral lead-in.

> **Doctor:** (To CA) "Mrs. Jones is right on schedule. Let's reduce her frequency as we discussed. In addition, on her next visit, she may be bringing her sister with her. Let's try to make her appointment at a time when I'll have a little extra time to talk with her."
>
> (To patient) "Mrs. Jones, I'll see you on Tuesday."

At that point, the doctor should turn and leave the front desk, letting the CA finish setting up the details of the next visit—scheduling new multiple appointments, presenting the appointment card, and booking time for the family member.

A last point to be made here, is that if the patient has young children who have not yet been brought to the office to have their spines checked for alteration of nerve flow caused by vertebral subluxations—they should. Approaching the subject of subluxation prevention and development care immediately after a successful reevaluation and re-consultation is only natural.

Remember, doing all of the right things, with the right intent for your patients will result in a high number parents who will gratefully bring their children in to be checked for subluxations. Timing is important in referral generation. Always be sensitive to the proper time, tone, and intent when discussing referrals with patients. The right words, spoken properly, with an attitude of compassion, personal mission, and noble intentions will allow you to fill your waiting room with entire families availing themselves of the miracles of health, wellness, and the opportunity to enhance their physical, mental, and emotional development.

Step 7-3: Keep Patients on Track— the Appointment Reminder Procedure

Missed appointments can be financially disastrous to the bottom line of a practice. Worse, they can be devastating to the ability of the patient to experience the best results possible under chiropractic care. Constantly trying to reduce the number of missed appointments should be the CA's personal charge. To reduce the number of missed appointments, the CA should call and confirm the appointments of patients who have set up appointments more than three weeks in advance. An effective alternative to the reminder telephone call is for the CA to e-mail the patient their reminder on the day preceding their appointment. This may be more effective and certainly more time efficient.

The reminder telephone call, however, is easy to accomplish. As the CA is pulling and dating the patient information cards for the next day's scheduled appointments, he or she should check the date of the patient's last visit. All patients with three weeks or greater interval between appointments should receive a telephone confirmation. Here, unlike the recall procedure, leaving a message on the patient's answering machine is okay. Such a simple procedure will drastically reduce the number of missed appointments.

CA: "Mrs. Jones? This is Carol from Dr. Meyer's office...I am calling to confirm your appointment tomorrow at (time of appointment)."

(If patient answers in the affirmative) "Thank you for your time, we'll see you tomorrow."

(If patient indicates they cannot make it) "I understand. Would you prefer that I reschedule you for later in the afternoon or for Friday?"

After speaking with the patient, record the fact that the patient was contacted in the appointment book. Patients' lives are extremely hectic, and those who are beginning to advance into health and wellness care can easily have their appointments "slip" their minds. Reminders keep patients on track and on schedule.

Step 7-4: Maintain Continuity— Forbid Missed Appointments

Unrescheduled missed appointments are one of the most common, yet least noticed ways patients may lose the continuity in their recommended program of care. As we discussed previously, missed appointments can be devastating to the patient's ability to experience the optimum benefits of chiropractic care. Therefore, it is critical to the patient's health and to practice stability that you have sound procedures and strict policies for both staff and patients on how to handle these situations. As in every aspect of office management, the doctor holds the final responsibility to ensure that patients are reappointed and that the importance of maintaining their schedule of care is strongly imprinted into the consciousness of every patient. Failure of the staff to reappoint patients who have missed their appointment is in direct proportion to the doctor's commitment to the patient's initial recommended program of care. In fact, when I see practices with high levels of missed appointments, I question the doctor's own commitment to his or her patients and practice. Look closely at your missed appointment rates. If they are greater than 10 percent, you need to ask yourself…how committed am I?

Besides the devastating effect that missed appointments have on the patient's ability to respond to their program of care, missed or canceled appointments account for the greatest drain on practice growth. Such a drain will dramatically impact financial stability of the practice more than any other aspect of its day-to-day operations. By multiplying the number of missed appointments by your office visit fee over a given time period, it is easy to demonstrate the financial loss to a practice because of missed appointments. Unfortunately, it is more difficult is to assess the resultant loss of a patient's progress if your recommendations and care regimen are not followed.

Staff Responsibility

It is the responsibility of the front desk CA to call and attempt to reschedule all missed appointments. There should be no questions and no excuses. But more importantly, it is the doctor's commitment to the patient that should keep him or her alert at all times as to whether the CA is keeping track of patients who miss appointments and is handling them effectively.

It is also the doctor's duty to the patient and the practice to take a hard-line approach with both the CA and the patient to see that all missed appointments are not only rescheduled, but also actually made up when missed.

Missed Appointment Log

WEEK ENDING ____/____/____

Name	Phone	Hm	Wk	Date Missed	Date Re-Schd	Contact Date	Pt. Ref.	Sched Error	PH By
1.									
2.									
3.									
4.									
5.									
6.									
7.									
8.									
9.									
10.									
11.									
12.									
13.									
14.									
15.									
16.									
17.									
18.									
19.									
20.									

Special Notes:

Sample Form: **Missed Appointment Log**

Make Up All Missed Appointments

Often, even the best patient will test you and your resolve in maintaining the recommended schedule of care. Because of the importance of consistency of care in assuring the anticipated patient response, the alteration of the preset multiple appointment schedules must not be allowed to occur. Therefore, all missed appointments should not only be rescheduled, but actually "made up" as well.

For example, if, in your professional opinion, your patient needs to be seen on a three-times-per-week basis, that patient might be scheduled for Monday, Wednesday, and Friday appointments. If the patient misses Monday's appointment, the patient should be contacted within 10 minutes of the missed appointment time, and all attempts to reschedule that patient for later that same day should be made.

If the patient is not able to reschedule the missed appointment on the same day it was missed, an effort should be made to reschedule and make up the appointment on the following day. If the patient insists they cannot make up that appointment on either of the days, the CA should politely remind them of their next regularly scheduled appointment and try to obtain a verbal commitment that the person will make that appointment.

When the patient does come in for their next regularly scheduled appointment, it then becomes the doctor's duty to reinforce the rationale for current recommendations and to insist that the patient return *before* the next regularly scheduled appointment to make up for the missed appointment.

With each missed appointment, the doctor's confidence and certainty in his or her technique and recommendations for clinical care, and in chiropractic are being tested. If the patient will not be held accountable for making up their missed appointments, the doctor cannot be held responsible for their health. I have always felt that patients who miss appointments or refuse to make up their missed appointment should be considered candidates for dismissal or referral. If they will not take responsibility for following the recommendations that they agreed to, I will not accept the responsibility of something as important as their health.

Benefits of "Making Up Missers"

The benefits of bringing the patient back on schedule and reinforcing their commitment to their health and comprehensive chiropractic care are threefold:

First, when patients are allowed to miss their appointments and to then merely continue on with the rest of their prearranged adjustments, those patients will either consciously or subconsciously believe the doctor was not all that committed to the course of care outlined for them at the outset. Steadfast recall procedures and making up missed appointments will confirm to the patient that the doctor and staff are committed. It shows that their doctor is serious about their doing what is in their best interest.

Also, by insisting that patients make up their missed appointments, the patient's rehabilitative and corrective progress can proceed as anticipated with ultimate results obtained. Failure to do so, may result in prolonged pain and disability, as well as necessitate added or prolonged care of that patient. Clearly, a missed appointment is a situation that is a detriment to the patient's health, and in the end, the doctor's reputation. The strongest argument for encouraging patients to make up missed appointments is that it not only enhances their chances of obtaining maximum results, but it also teaches the offending patients they will be confronted and held accountable for any future missed appointments. This will cause them to think twice before they miss another.

Finally, as discussed earlier, when missed appointments are not rescheduled or made up, significant income will be lost to the practice. Over the course of the year, this loss may total thousands of dollars. Worse, missed appointments will cause you to be far less productive and prevent other patients from being able to schedule needed appointments during these times. Using a hard-line approach about missed appointments will lead to improved office and doctor efficiency.

Conclusion

When you and your staff insist on patients making up appointments that are missed during their initial phases of care, the patient will quickly realize that you are sincere and dedicated to the original course of care that was outlined and accepted. The patient will come to know that you are committed to seeing that recommendations are followed, and that they obtain the absolute best results possible by correcting their vertebral subluxation complex.

Although this policy may take some backbone to enforce, is not difficult for either you or the CA. But, it is ultimately up to the doctor to make the effort and to have the courage to insist that the patient follows the prescribed clinical course of chiropractic care. If rescheduling and making up missed appointments is accomplished on a routine basis, the benefit realized by both the patient and the practice makes that extra effort pay off in a big way, in both improved clinical results and greater financial rewards for the practice.

After almost three decades of managing my staff, my patients, and my practices, I have learned that an important step on the "stairway to success" is to understand that practice success is often a "shedding" process. It is the releasing or referring of patients who will not or cannot accept your practice paradigm or who become consistent sources of stress to your practice. I recommend that you release patients who are wasting your time. You will be amazed at how liberating it is, and how once these patients have left your practice you will have room and energies for many others who will surely take their place. Please, doctors, spend your energies on those who want what you and your practice have to offer—not on catering to and babysitting those who do not.

Step 7-5: "Out of Sight" Must Never Be "Out of Mind"—Patient Recall

I maintain that the best patient to have is the patient you have! Therefore, patient recall is a tremendously beneficial procedure for assuring the future health and well-being of all patients—and your practice. In most cases, preventative measures can prove effective in saving patients time, money, and most importantly, needless pain and suffering.

The most effective recall procedure is that which is accomplished face-to-face with the patient at the end of each office visit—the rescheduling of the next appointment. To be successful, the doctor and the front desk staff must work together to impress upon the patient the importance of follow-up care when indicated. The effectiveness of scheduling needed future visits at the end of each visit will greatly aid in reducing the amount of inactive patient recall. While the motivation and education for patients' understanding their healthcare and making the right decision always rests squarely on the shoulders of the doctor, the execution lies with the CA.

In *every* case, at the end of *every* visit, the doctor should tell *every* patient when to return. And to explain and to reinforce with them the reason why. It is surprising to most doctors to learn that the majority of their patients actually want to be told how to take care of themselves. Such instructions are vital to the continued proper decision making of the patient, and therefore, their continued well-being. To communicate the patient's need for follow-up care, the doctor must be sure that the length of time between appointments is noted on the patient's receipt or travel slip before the patient is released to the CA at the end of each visit.

After the doctor releases the patient, it is important for the CA to effectively follow up and schedule the next appointment before the patient leaves the office. Proper booking techniques that were described earlier are the best way to prevent patients from leaving the office without a future appointment.

Remember, when scheduling a new appointment, the CA must never give the patient a choice of only one date or time. As we discussed previously, if the patient refuses a single time offering, the CA is trapped into continuing to repeat the procedure again and again, until he or she can get the patient to accept a specific time. Such a procedure is always time-consuming, frustrating, and unproductive for both staff and patient.

It is much more efficient for the CA to give the patient a choice between days and times that he or she wishes to have filled as the block-booking procedure dictates. Offering an "either/or" choice appears to allow the patient make the decision as to their next appointment, but at the same time, the CA is retaining the ability to direct the flow of appointments and properly block-book, making the schedule effective and efficient.

> **CA:** "Mrs. Jones, you will want to have that checked in a month. Would Tuesday the 12th or Thursday the 14th be better? Morning or afternoon?"

Often when the practice is extremely busy and the staff has other pressing needs, it may seem easier to just tell patients they are due back in three weeks and to let them leave without taking time to actually schedule another appointment. Such a casual approach is not only devastating for the practice, but it is a great disservice to the patient as well. Even with good intentions, the patient may get busy and forget to call for an appointment. One of the most important rules of the office should be: "Every effort should be made by the CA to schedule a subsequent appointment before the patient leaves."

Again, there is one point in this entire procedure that cannot be made strongly enough. It is the doctor's responsibility to tell the patient *when* to return and *why*. Then, the doctor must get the patient's commitment before allowing him or her to leave the adjusting room. Reinforcing the specific objectives of care, the patient's status or progress, and a reminder of subsequent objectives to be reached does this quite effectively and with a low level of confrontation.

> **Doctor:** "Mrs. Jones, your spine is beginning to stabilize nicely but it still has a way to go. You will need to have that checked and probably adjusted again at the end of the week. That way, we can prevent you from drifting back to where you started."

It is the CA's job to reschedule the appointment—never to pressure the patient into making it. Some patients, however, may periodically (or routinely) decline to make further appointments. A large percentage of this group are patients who only return when they are symptomatic. Some may simply have scheduling difficulties. Young mothers, truck drivers, and busy business people who travel and do not know their schedules weeks in advance will often fall into this category.

Quite frequently, patients who fall into this group will say: "Let me check my schedule and call you back."

Such a situation can be handled this way:

> **CA:** "Just in case the appointment book fills up, I will hold a 10:00 A.M. on Tuesday for you. When you know your schedule, can you call me back if this does not work?"

If the patient still declines to make an appointment, the CA should place the patient's name, phone number, and day of appointment on a slip of paper and call the person back within the next few days to reschedule the next appointment once his or her schedule is known.

Patient Recall and Recapture Procedure

From time to time, the doctor will advise a patient to return for a follow-up visit whenever the *patient* feels the need. Generally the doctor will indicate this by putting the initials RAN (return as needed) on the patient's service slip. Then, the doctor will write "5 weeks," "7 weeks," etc. on the slip. In such an instance, the patient's name and phone number should be entered into the patient recall book for future recall at the above time intervals.

Step 7-6: Understand Your Patients—Maintain Control

Frustrating as it may be, every practice has its share of "uncontrollable" patients. These are those patients who, for their own reasons, will not follow your recommendations, office policies, or just cause stress in the practice. Fortunately, these patients always fall into six distinct categories. Once recognized and placed in a proper category, these patients may be dealt with appropriately. Some can be salvaged and turned into great patients, others should be dismissed from your practice, thereby making room for the patients upon whom you will build your ideal practice.

Study the following and learn to recognize them. Recognition of a problem is the first step toward solving it.

1. The "Uncontrollable" Patient. The "uncontrollable" patient is often someone who has received "treatment" in another chiropractic office. They usually come into the office dictating to you what they want and what they don't want as far a care and case management. Usually, they misguidedly see chiropractic as an expensive but effective aspirin. They only want an adjustment to afford them temporary relief and will not bother with proper correction. Quite often these patients will refuse to make another appointment or, if they are not symptomatic, will not keep appointments they do make. Even worse, when this type of patient does arrive at their appointment, they are often late and will complain about having to wait.

◆ Keep Your Patients Educated, Excited, and Adjusted ◆

The proper solution for this type of patient depends on the kind of practice you wish to have. If these patients do not fit the paradigm of your practice, you must be honest and forthright with the patient and discuss these problems with them. These patients do not understand or realize their actions are not in keeping with the practice that you are trying to design; they only understand their model of chiropractic. Unfortunately, they were introduced to this model by a previous chiropractor who may not have understood or communicated the concept of relief, correction, and stabilization of the vertebral subluxation complex.

For your own sanity, and the patient's own good, you must sit down with the patient and explain to them the nature of the vertebral subluxation complex and how it impacts his or her health concerns. Also, you must describe the type of practice you are trying to build and the benefits of remaining a patient in this type of practice. Then, you may invite the patient to become a valued member of your practice. Often, after such a discussion, the patient will "see the light" and may become one of your most conscientious patients.

If not, and the patient simply reiterates he or she just wants a "pop in the neck," you should gently and respectfully help them to understand they simply do not fit into the parameters of the type of patient you wish to take care of. At that point, you may offer to refer the "uncontrollable" patient to another practice in your area that embraces this type of patient.

It has been my experience on more than one occasion that following just such a discussion (especially if the doctor offers to make a referral), such patients see the doctor's commitment to building a quality practice and will "buy into" the chiropractic vision of health and wellness. Such patients will actually, almost magically, transform themselves into the ideal patient. If such an awakening occurs, you should get the patient's commitment to follow your recommendations and all other expectations that you have of your patients.

Again, I believe that success is the "pruning out" of patients who do not fit your paradigm of chiropractic. While we all would like care for every patient who enters our office, sometimes we need to refer patients to allow our practice to grow. It seems that for every patient we release back to the universe, we create openings for others who are searching for the type of care we have to offer. You must constantly strive to never fill your practice with frustrating patients. If they frustrate you, the odds are good that you also frustrate them.

If the patient cannot agree to your chiropractic, health, and practice vision, and to your policies and procedures, you must then dismiss the patient from care. Appropriately discussed, and a referral to another practice made, the patient should leave with both a deeper understanding and greater goodwill toward you and your practice.

2. "Will Call" Patients. The "will call" patient is often a long-standing patient in your office, someone who has followed your recommendations, been a model patient, but for many reasons cannot or will not schedule their next appointment. They may also be a patient who knows when they need to return and can be relied upon to call when necessary.

These are patients who, like the "uncontrollable," call for care when they feel the need. However, unlike the "uncontrollable," do not wait too long after realizing that they need to "get checked" to come into the office. The "will call" patient is usually a good patient. They are usually on time and seldom miss their appointments. They understand the role of staying adjusted and having their subluxations corrected before they become symptomatic. "Will call" patients are sometimes among your favorite patients, but rather than making appointments in advance, they call for care on an as-needed basis.

Many successful practices are filled with this type of patient. Here, you should continually reinforce the need for return visits when they are indicated for these patients. It is best for you to make a "WC" (will call) notation on the receipt, followed by time-interval recommendation for the next visit. In such a case, the CA should record the patient's name and phone number in the appointment book at noted intervals and call the patient to remind him or her of the need for their next appointment.

3. "Canceled Appointment—Can't Reschedule" Patient. This patient is usually a current or active patient who is in one of the various stages of condition-based care. Typically, they cancel a scheduled (or multiple appointment program) appointment because of an emergency or a conflict, and simply advise the CA they will call later. Unless handled properly, these may be the biggest group of patients lost to a practice. In many cases a legitimate situation has arisen where it is necessary for the patient to cancel; in other cases, the patient may simply be trying to drop out of care in a nonconfrontational manner.

In either case, the CA should record the patient's name and phone number in the appointment book. Then, one or two weeks later, he or she should call the patient to reschedule the appointment. If the patient does reschedule, it is the CA's responsibility to review the patient's multiple appointment schedule and revise it if necessary. It is also important that you, as the doctor, are aware of these situations and deal with them appropriately.

4. "Vacation" Patients. A "vacation" patient is a regular patient in any phase of care who cancels or cannot schedule an appointment because of an upcoming vacation or business trip. Keeping track of these patients is vital in preventing patient attrition. Whenever a patient cancels an appointment or does not schedule because of an approaching trip, the CA should ascertain when the patient is scheduled to return. The CA should then record the patient's return a few days past the date in the appointment book and later phone the patient to reschedule their appointment.

5. "Nonprogrammed" New Patients. From time to time, you may have new patients enter your practice who have all of the characteristics of an ideal patient; they have chosen relief, correction, stabilization, and will ultimately select to avail themselves to the benefits of long-term wellness care. They are serious about their health and sincere about getting the recommended chiropractic care. But, when the CA attempts to create a case management plan for them, they discover that their work, schedule, or lifestyle simply does not allow them to commit themselves to a specific time or day. This is quite common in local delivery truck drivers and others whose occupations prevent any type of set schedule.

Unfortunately, these patients must be appointed on a visit-to-visit basis. In such cases, it is difficult for all concerned to actually keep track of where the patient is as they progress through their care. To help record their progress through the recommended period of care, and to know when reevaluations are due, the CA should mark the days of anticipated visits on the patient information card, noting that appointments must be made at each visit as they progress through their recommended schedule. It is then up to the doctor to follow the case management calendar on the patient information card, and then advise and reinforce the appointments to the patient on an ongoing basis.

To reinforce the next visit and the need for the front desk to re-schedule, it is important that the doctor write the day of the patient's next visit on the service slip so that the CA will know when to schedule the patient for their next adjustment.

6. "Leaves Office Without Appointment." This patient is not so "uncontrollable" as forgetful. They have simply failed to make a follow-up appointment at the last visit. This is just as much the fault of the CA as it is the patient. This most commonly happens to longtime patients who have gotten friendly with the staff and are prone to engage the CA in extraneous conversation, letting the follow-up appointment slip in the process. For whatever reason, this patient simply gets out of the office without setting a new appointment time.

In this situation, once the CA realizes the mistake, he or she should merely set the patient's card aside. Then, within the hour, the CA can telephone the patient to schedule the next appointment.

Step 7-7: Getting a Second Chance—Managing Returning Inactive Patients

Patients Not Seen in Six Months or Longer

As we discussed earlier, the appearance of an undetected and unexpected new patient will destroy your schedule, because of the length of time needed to process this patient properly. In the same manner, an undetected and unexpected patient whose record is not up-to-date or who presents with a new health concern will pose exactly the same problems to an unprepared, unsuspecting staff.

Unlike the new patient, the returning inactive patient (RIP) may pose even greater problems. Many times, RIPs may present with a totally different set of complaints, have had an accident or injury, or such time has passed that their entire health picture has changed.

It is important that the front desk CA (or anyone answering the telephone) always knows the exact status of each person calling for an appointment. The following procedures are required in any situation where the front desk CA does not immediately recognize the caller.

Patient Status Determination

This procedure is exactly like the procedure used in determining the new patient. If the CA does not immediately recognize the caller's name, or if he or she does...and realizes that it has been quite a while since that patient has been in the office, the CA should politely ask the patient:

CA: "Mrs. Jones, when was the last time you saw the doctor?"

> *Note:* If it has been over six months, or the date of the last appointment is in question, the CA must immediately pull the patient's card and verify the length of time since the last visit.

CA: "Mrs. Jones, would you pardon me just one moment while I pull your file?"

The CA should try to determine if the visit will take any longer than average for a returning patient. By asking the following questions he or she will get a good idea as to how to book the patient. A perfect way to do this is to complete the health information update section of the established patient update form *before* offering the patient an appointment.

CA: "Okay, Mrs. Jones, what is your major complaint at this time?"

"How severe is this complaint?

"How long have you had this problem?

"Are you having any other health concerns?

"Have you had any falls, accidents, or been to another doctor since you were last in our office?"

Once the CA has obtained the necessary information, he or she may continue to book the patient, allowing enough time for the patient to be re-consulted and possibly reexamined and re-x-rayed. If your consultation procedures are efficient, and the exam well-designed, this procedure should take no more than 15 to 20 minutes to complete.

"Returning Inactive Patient" Processing

Once the returning inactive patient has entered the office for an appointment, he or she should be treated exactly like a new patient. The patient should be asked to have a seat, given an established patient update form, a patient financial options form, and an informed consent form. The patient should then be taken to the consultation/examination room—not to the adjusting room.

The patient will then be re-consulted by the doctor and, if necessary, reexamined and re-x-rayed. The CA should always remember that the decision to reexamine or re-x-ray is the decision of the doctor, and that it is based solely on the clinical presentation of the patient. The CA should never imply to the patient that there will be anything out of the routine for the visit. Should the patient inquire as to the need for the new forms to be filled out, the CA will merely respond that it is a file update. Any decisions to be made as to how to proceed with the patient on a clinical level is the doctor's responsibility after he or she has had a chance to update the patient's consultation and history. It is the CA's responsibility to identify the returning inactive patient and to schedule accordingly.

Remember, this individual has been a patient before, maybe a good patient, maybe not so good. However, somewhere, somehow, they did not get the message about the subluxation complex, normal function and adaptation, health, chiropractic, and true wellness. This, doctor, is a rare second chance to reeducate the patient and restate your chiropractic message. This time you may actually be able to help this individual lead a better life by understanding and choosing to live subluxation-free.

Once the patient has completed their forms, the patient should be escorted to the consultation room for the doctor to update the patient's file. There may be nothing extra to be done, other than to simply adjust the patient. But, in all cases, appropriate time should be reserved just in case the patient presents with a different clinical picture.

The "established patient update form" is similar to the new patient information form. It is designed to gather the necessary patient information on patients who have not been seen in some time, without generating a protest by the patient that this information was already provided when he or she initially entered the practice. It also helps the

◆ Keep Your Patients Educated, Excited, and Adjusted ◆

Established Patient Update

Welcome!	**Welcome Back!** Since it has been several months since your last visit to our office, we must verify that our records are still accurate and up-to-date. Please take a few minutes and complete the following. It is important that the doctor knows of any changes that might impact on the care that you will receive. *Thank You.*
Personal Information Update	Name:_____ Address / Phone: ☐ Same ☐ New:_____ _____ Employer: ☐ Same ☐ New:_____ Work Activities:_____ Current Hobbies / Sports:_____

Health Information Update	Current complaint:_____
	
	How severe is this complaint? ☐ Mild ☐ Moderate ☐ Severe
	
	Is this complaint the result of a fall, accident, or work related injury?
	☐ Yes ☐ No If "Yes" Please Explain:_____
	_____.
	
	Since your last visit to this office, have you:
	    Had any falls or accidents? ☐ Yes ☐ No
	    Had any fractures or broken bones? ☐ Yes ☐ No
	    Been hospitalized? ☐ Yes ☐ No
	    Seen any other doctor? ☐ Yes ☐ No
	
	If yes to any of the above, please give details:_____
	_____
	_____
	_____

Sample Form: **Established Patient Update (front)**

Established Patient Update (Side 2)

Check Any Of The Following That May Apply To You

Health Issues:
- ☐ Polio
- ☐ Cancer
- ☐ Diabetes
- ☐ High Stress
- ☐ Under Weight
- ☐ Arthritis
- ☐ AIDS or ARC
- ☐ Frequent Illnesses
- ☐ Poor Diet
- ☐ Other:_____
- ☐ Diabetes
- ☐ Heart
- ☐ Allergies
- ☐ Epilepsy
- ☐ Sleeplessness
- ☐ Chronic Fatigue
- ☐ Genetic Disorders
- ☐ Over Weight

Intake Or Use:
- ☐ Alcohol
- ☐ Sleeping Pills
- ☐ Tobacco
- ☐ Other:_____
- ☐ Pain Relievers
- ☐ Caffiene

Check Any Problems That You May Have Had Within The Past Six Months

Muscles—Skeleton
- ☐ Low Back Pain
- ☐ Middle Back
- ☐ Neck
- ☐ Shoulders / Arms
- ☐ Joint Pain / Stiffness
- ☐ Hips / Legs

Nerve System
- ☐ Headaches
- ☐ Nervousness
- ☐ Numbness / Tingling
- ☐ Muscle Weakness
- ☐ Dizziness
- ☐ Forgetfulness
- ☐ Depression
- ☐ Fainting
- ☐ Seizures
- ☐ Cold Hands / Feet
- ☐ Stress Reactions
- ☐ Shaking / Tremors

Circulation—Breathing
- ☐ Chest
- ☐ Lungs / Breathing
- ☐ Blood Pressure
- ☐ Heart Rate
- ☐ Chest Pain
- ☐ Sinus Pain

Digestion—Elimination
- ☐ Poor Appetite
- ☐ Excessive Thirst
- ☐ Nausea
- ☐ Diarrhea
- ☐ Constipation
- ☐ Hemorrhoids
- ☐ Weight Loss / Gain
- ☐ Heartburn
- ☐ Change In Stools

Eye—Ear—Nose—Throat
- ☐ Eyes / Vision
- ☐ Dental / TMJ
- ☐ Throat / Voice
- ☐ Ears / Hearing
- ☐ Sinus
- ☐ Circulation

Urinary—Genitals
- ☐ Pain With Urination
- ☐ Infrequent Urination
- ☐ Frequent Urination
- ☐ Weak Stream
- ☐ Bladder Control
- ☐ Genitals

Female Only
- ☐ Menstrual
- ☐ Low Back W/ Per.
- ☐ Pain With Urination
- ☐ Breast

Are You Pregnant? ☐ Yes ☐ No

Please Mark Area Of Concern

(X) Pain
(O) Spasm
(-) Numb

I understand that my care in this office may involve the making of judgements that are based upon the facts known by the doctor. Therfore, the above information is true and complete to the best of my knowledge. I also understand that the practice of any healing art is not an exact science and that no guarantee of results will be made by the doctor nor relied upon by me. I furhter understand that the doctor's professional expertise lies in detecting and correcting the structural and mechanical abberations of the spine - the Vertebral Subluxation Complex. I agree that I will not hold the doctor responsible for the diagnosis or treatment of any medical condition indicated above.

Patient's Signature:

Sample Form: **Established Patient Update (front)**

doctor and staff to keep all of the patient's personal files up-to-date. The reverse side of the form is the same as the new patient information form, and once filled out should be compared carefully with the original. In a busy office, the CA can scan for any changes prior to the doctor's seeing the patient. He or she may then highlight any differences to alert the doctor to any possible changes. With all of the needed updated information, the doctor can now properly determine how he or she wishes to manage the patient on a clinical level.

Key Points

- Only by utilizing objective and subjective reevaluations can the doctor and patient have a true perspective of the attainment of the objectives of proper management.

- Periodic reevaluations and comparative reviews must be used as the foundation of all ethical patient management procedures.

- An effective means to evaluate the patient's subjective reports is to use a visual analog scale that renders a numerical value to their complaints during the initial consultation and at the time of re-evaluation. It should be emphasized that the comparative report should be done with seriousness and high intention, that is, with both energy and importance. This is one of the most critical components of patient case management.

- The symptoms of the vertebral subluxation complex will often resolve long before the underlying correction has taken place.

- If the patient has completed the initial three objectives of the condition-based care and all objective findings of the subluxation complex have been significantly resolved, the patient will be classified as a wellness patient.

- The family health history form now becomes an excellent source of information about family members who may have or be developing subluxations and resultant health problems that chiropractic can effectively address.

Bonus Solution 1

Generate New Patient Referrals

A successful practice should never have to resort to long-term advertising or gimmicks and giveaways to attract new patients. A practice that is well-conceived, established, and managed with the right philosophies and the right principles, and that provides high quality care with an attitude of loving service, will be an oasis people will want to come to and tell their friends about. There are many ways to market your practice and to attract new patients, but the easiest and most cost-effective way for an established practice is through referrals.

In this section, your first "bonus solution" to practice success, we will discuss how you can stimulate referrals by simply assisting your patients in their efforts to fill your office with their family and friends. If you are looking for an easy, cheap, foolproof, yet ethical "gimmick" that will fill your practice with quality patients, I will tell you that I do not know of any nor do I believe one exists.

I do know that if you are willing to work hard and go the extra mile for your patients, the following systems to stimulate quality referrals are inexpensive, foolproof, and ethical. They will, however, require effort and motivation.

I have saved this section on referrals for last because implementing the previous policies and procedures we have discussed will set the stage for developing each new patient into a lifelong, referring chiropractic patient. Attracting new patients without having the other policies and procedures we have discussed in place is a tragedy. Those encouraged to become patients in a chiropractic office not procedurally ready for them will stay for a short time—if at all. They will not get the long-term lasting results that chiropractic offers, and will prematurely evaporate from the practice.

Not only is this not the way to build your practice, but also it is a grave disservice to those unfortunate people who sought your care. Oh, maybe their clinical care was up to par, or even superb, but they were not educated and cared for in a way that would bring them into the fold of lifetime "wellness" patients. As a result, they may think chiropractic is merely a "treatment" for symptoms…or even a "treatment" for subluxations. But they were not brought to the point where they realize the astounding health and life-enhancing promise of living life subluxation-free.

Therefore, before you begin to attract large volumes of referred new patients, you must ask yourself the following questions: "Have I designed the appropriate policies and procedures to properly manage my practice and patients so they will avail themselves of proper care in my office?" "Have I developed the staff that I dreamed of in Solution 2?" "Are my policies, systems, forms, and scripts in place?" If so, you are now ready to fill your practice with prospective ideal patients. Read on.

Bonus Step 1-1: Develop a Referral Atmosphere

Essential to the growth of any practice is the adequate infusion of new patients. The number of new patients needed must equal the number of those lost to the normal attrition of already established patients as well as generate sufficient numbers to account for the desired rate of practice growth.

The procurement of new patients is not a magical, mystical procedure, but merely the end result of proper office procedures: providing positive clinical results and caring for your patients as you would want your own family cared for.

New patients can come from three primary sources:

1. Referrals—Referred new patients are those generated by established patients who are both satisfied with and enthusiastic about the doctor, the office, and the procedures, or by employers and other persons of influence who are impressed with your practice reputation and your ability to effect positive clinical results.

2. Advertising—Some new patients are attracted to the office by outside advertising or promotions, such as newspapers, media, and screenings or direct mailings. This may also include the doctor's self-promotion and visibility in the community.

3. Off the street—This patient appears to choose your office at random because of its location or because of a listing in the Yellow Pages, signage, etc.

While advertising and accepting walk-in patients may be necessary during the first few years of practice in order to build your base, an established practice should not have to rely on these sources for new patients or practice growth. For our purposes, we will ignore those sources of new patients that are either expensive or uncontrollable (advertising and off the street). Here we will concentrate on encouraging and enabling your existing patients to refer to you. Hopefully, by promoting your practice as we discussed earlier you will never need an advertising campaign. Off-the-street patients will be a nice bonus to add to your eventual list of overflow patients, but consistently generating patient referrals is a predictable and controllable way to attract quality new patients and build the practice of your dreams.

Bonus Step 1-2: Consciously Implement Referral Strategies

To work effectively, the referral procedures that attract new patients are well-designed strategies the doctor must be conscious of implementing at all times. Properly executed, these procedures hold the promise of securing the greatest volume of new patients, in a predictable manner, while adding nothing to your overhead.

The number of new patients who come into your office under this category is the best indication of your ability to interact properly with the patient, the staff's efficiency, and sound office procedures. However, groundwork must be laid to enhance the effectiveness of these strategies. The following are prerequisites before a patient can or will want to refer friends, relatives, and acquaintances to you.

Strategy One: Utilize the "Law of Obligation"

If you want to motivate your patients to work for you, you must create an environment where the patient feels "obliged" to help you to build your practice and fulfill your destiny in life. How in the world can you do this? In simple words: Make them feel so good about you and your office that they will either consciously or subconsciously feel obligated to give something back to you in order for them to reach a position of "even exchange."

To accomplish this mutually beneficial situation is both easy and fun. Yes, it can even become a great game. Simply, you and your staff must find ways to give your patients more empathy, understanding, consideration, concern, love, recognition, appreciation, and clinical results than they have ever experienced from a professional practice. In short, the patient must feel they have received more than they expected and certainly more than they paid for.

In other words, you and your staff must do more for the patient than any other doctor has ever done under similar circumstances. Doing so will make the patient both excited about being in your practice, and enthusiastic about referring others to your practice. Remember though while creating such an environment in your office is fun and exciting, "obligation" is a powerful motivator. You must always remember that you are using this tremendous concept because caring for your patients in this manner is the right thing to do. It is how you would like to be treated and certainly how you would like your loved ones to be treated. But, at the same time you must recognize the impact such care will have on a patient's desire to reciprocate in an acceptable and appropriate manner.

♦ Generate New Patient Referrals ♦

Remember what we said earlier:

> Making a patient enthusiastic,
> NOT
> merely satisfied
> is the key to referrals.

This process is called the law of obligation, and occurs when patients realize that at every point of patient-doctor-staff interactions, their expectations have been exceeded. For instance, when a patient comes into the office, receives and pays for an examination, or gets and pays for an adjustment, an equal rate of exchange takes place and your relationship with your patient is in balance; you owe the patient nothing, and the patient owes you nothing.

If, on the other hand, the patient receives the expected care, pays you for your services, but then you continue to do many little extra services, show extra concern, provide outstanding service—in short, give them more than they expect or more than they pay you for, they will remain out of exchange with you. You have done more for them than they have done for you. A patient in this situation will subconsciously strive to regain an even rate of exchange.

These extra services and concerns may include some of the following:

- Calling new and acute patients the afternoon or evening after they have been adjusted.
- Sending them thank-you letters for referrals.
- Giving more of you to the patient than they expect (e.g., in-depth examinations, complete consultation, present-time consciousness, regular in-depth examinations, etc.).
- Giving out business cards with the doctor's home phone number handwritten on the back, while telling the patient you are always available for them in case of an emergency.
- Sending personal welcome notes to new patients. (Handwritten is best.)
- When patients are spread out to one full week between appointments, having a staff member contact them about midweek to inquire as to how they are getting along.

- Sending your patients personally signed birthday cards.
- Loving your patient. Seeing and caring for each patient as if that person were your spouse, mother, father, brother, sister, or child.
- Providing a spinal-care class to teach patients how to enhance their care.

The number of added services that can create higher and higher levels of unequal exchange and patient obligation is limited only by your imagination. A wonderful agenda item for staff meetings might be for the doctor and staff to brainstorm and to come up with many more ideas that will ultimately lead to the desired results. You might discuss who may have come into negative exchange with your practice since the last staff meeting, and the "who" and "how" that was accomplished. Exploring new ideas to apply the law of obligation at your staff meetings makes them fun and exciting.

Typically, chiropractic offices intentionally or unintentionally apply this law to some degree. However, most practices do not go far enough to reap the rewards of their efforts, because the patients do not know how to "get even." Most doctors and staff think their patients are psychic and should be able to know that if they want to thank us for our efforts they should refer patients to our practice. Patients are not psychic; they have no idea you wish to serve more patients and that you would love them even more if they sent you their friends and family. Provided you and your staff can do all of the above, you must now channel the patient's efforts toward the desired end of regaining a balanced exchange by referring new patients to your practice.

Strategy Two: Create Conditions That Allow for Patient Referrals

Before a patient can comfortably refer to you, you must meet certain conditions that will encourage the patient to naturally refer others to your practice:

- The patient must be made aware that you have the time and the desire to help more people. The best way to accomplish this is to routinely be on time, attentive to the patient, talk only about the patient's concerns (health and chiropractic). The doctor must never discuss "interests" such as sports, weather, etc.

- The patient must have no doubts that you are skilled, competent, professional, principled, and that you really care about your patients. Remember the old saying: "The patient doesn't really care how much you know for them to refer their friends and family, the patient has to know how much you care."
- Project the same or higher socioeconomic level as the referring patient. Remember, patients will find it difficult to refer others from their social status to a doctor who projects a lower socioeconomic level. Grooming, dress, speech and vocabulary, and mannerisms all speak loudly of who you are. Always dress well in the office, be clean, in good physical condition, speak well, and project an aura of professionalism. This holds just as true for your staff.
- The patient must be satisfied with the healthcare they receive in your office before they will encourage their friends and loved ones to come under your care. Your adjustments must be gentle yet effective, your clinical procedures thorough, and your knowledge apparent. Most importantly, you must project an air of clinical and personal certainty. You must have no doubts that chiropractic care is appropriate and effective. In addition you must own a sense of certainty that you have the ability to deliver. Almost as important, the patient must be satisfied with the responsiveness and the efficiency of the staff.
- You must be enthusiastic, positive, never be a "downer." Remember, your practice may be the only oasis of warmth and understanding the patient may encounter in their life. Strive to make their visit a fun, optimistic, and uplifting experience. Work to eliminate any discussion about current events, which tend to be depressing. Talk of hope and anticipation of when the patient will regain their health.
- Always operate in the present, that is, you must always be mentally concentrating on the patient you are with. You must project a high level of sincere interest in that patient and their family. This means you must practice mental discipline. You must strive to put the previous patient out of your mind; don't think about the upcoming ball game, the weather; or any personal difficulties you may be dealing with. Concentrate on your present patient and the subluxation

and resultant subluxation complex that brought this person to your office.

- Be personable, yet authoritative. The first thing you must realize is that you cannot socialize your way to success. The more you visit with your patients, the more you work at socializing and becoming a personal friend, the less effective you become as a healer. You must, above all else, avoid "chit-chatting" with your patients about things that are not pertinent to the reason the patient is in your office. If you can remain on the pedestal of professionalism, prevent personal familiarity with the patient, and maintain the role of an authority figure, patients will be much more likely to feel comfortable referring their friends to you and your practice. I am certain the less the patient knows about you on a personal level, the more they will follow your recommendations, and the more they will refer.

- You must ask for referrals. The very moment the patient begins expressing positive results from chiropractic care, they are at that instant, the most open for you and you staff to ask for referrals. This is the time you might utilize the family health history or the referral request procedure (described later) to stimulate referrals.

- Hold regular healthcare classes. Strongly urge (even require) your patients to attend your spinal-care class and specifically invite them to bring a friend, relative, or spouse. Remind them on each visit prior to the class of its importance in their long-term care. Hint to them about some of the information that will be given. To be most successful, your enthusiasm about the class will provide the impetus for patients to attend.

Bonus Step 1-3: Double Your Referral Sources—Spouses at the Case Report

The presence of the spouse at the case report serves to familiarize the spouse with both you and with chiropractic. By attending the case report, the spouse understands why his or her mate is in ill health, thus helping the spouse to be more sympathetic, understanding, and encouraging. At this time also, the spouse will be given the opportunity to understand why the patient will need to be seen on a regular basis and what the clinical objectives are in managing the case. Quite often this simple strategy will transform the spouse into a valuable ally rather than a nonunderstanding skeptic and detractor.

Of even greater benefit, the husband or wife now becomes more knowledgeable about chiropractic, and may become a patient or, at least, become a source of referrals.

At each case report (when the spouse is present) you should explain the healthcare class and make a special point to invite the spouse to attend as well. The point should be made that since the spouse lives in the same house, sleeps in the same bed, rides in the same car, sits in the same furniture, etc. they may be subject to the same spinal stressors as well. When the spouse is made aware that, in many cases, lifestyle sets the stage for many spinal-related problems, the spouse may begin to understand the wisdom of attending the class. You may also offer to examine the spouse at no charge after the class, thus setting the stage for an easy referral.

If you have done a good job with your patient leading up to this point, the spouse will be receptive to this idea, and the patient will usually encourage the spouse to follow through.

After the ensuing first adjustment, you may simply walk the new patient and the spouse to the front desk and instruct the CA to schedule an appointment for the patient's spouse after the healthcare class, and to give him or her a complimentary examination card.

Using this method alone, your new patient volume has just doubled.

Bonus Step 1-4: Stimulate Referrals from Your Healthcare Classes

A healthcare class is the single greatest practice builder known to the chiropractic profession. It is a practice builder only because it is a way and a means to continue to serve your patients. Here is your opportunity to help the patient and his or her spouse better understand chiropractic, as well as provide valuable information so they will become better patients.

A properly designed, well-delivered class will indeed show your patients how much you care about their health and the health of their families. Setting an evening aside to enhance their knowledge of chiropractic and teach them how to get well faster and stay well is value-added service as well as simply going the extra mile. Such a service will, of course, upset the balance of exchange that was mentioned earlier, creating an environment for further referrals.

By the time that you have finished with the class, given of your time, your knowledge, and your enthusiasm, your patients should be ready to do almost anything you ask in an effort to repay you. The exciting aspect about a healthcare class is that you never ask your patient to do anything for you at all. In fact, at the end of each class, you will offer to perform even more services to your patients by extending an invitation for complimentary consultations and examinations to their friends, families, and loved ones.

Here, the only thing that is asked of patients in return is for him or her to give you the chance to further fulfill your practice's mission by serving them even more. Following up on this invitation is still the responsibility of both you and your staff.

The best prospect is the nonpatient who has attended your healthcare class. To further encourage them to have their spines examined, you must require that the friends and family members in attendance sign up for their complimentary examinations before leaving the class. This is most effective if a class sign-in sheet is circulated prior to the beginning of the class. This will give the CA the names of those in attendance. During the class, the CA must prepare complimentary cards to be given to these people. Then at the end of the class the cards may be given to the person when they schedule their appointment.

Complimentary examinations that are requested for anyone not in attendance will require you to give the cards to the patient on a subsequent visit. Here the CA should have them prepared in advance and clipped to the patient's chart. After the patient's adjustment, you should perform an in absentia consultation about the prospective new patient. After discussing the case with the patient, you must walk with patient to the front desk, and encourage them to make appointments for the people they signed up prior to leaving the office.

As you can see, the stimulation of in-house new patients is simply a matter of doing everything right from the minute that person walks into your office. Doing more for your patients than they expect or require puts the patients in the proper position to work diligently for you and help you to build the practice of your dreams. All you must do is channel the patient's efforts toward the desired result of helping you to fill your practice with patients.

Work initially at developing and refining the previous procedures. Try to incorporate them into your daily practice routine. Eventually, these procedures will become automatic, and you will find yourself with an endless abundance of new patients.

Bonus Step 1-5: Explore the Genetic Link— the Well-Adjusted Family

The family health history form that the patient completes after their first visit is vital for five basic reasons. Most importantly, it will quickly and effortlessly provide you with information that will give valuable clinical insight into the patient's family background and the familial predisposition for spinal characteristics that caused them to seek chiropractic care. The patient's condition may be caused or predisposed by a genetic fault or familial trait leading to such problems. This being the case, the information from the family health history form may have a significant impact on the type of care rendered, as well as the clinical management of the case.

Second, if the patient is subjected to considerable destructive lifestyle circumstances, members of the immediate family may also be at risk for similar problems, especially if their spouse has similar complaints. Lifestyle and habits are an important area to investigate to more thoroughly help the patient and stimulate referrals. Suggestions for lifestyle changes may be an important concern in the management of such a case.

Third, should a strong family background of similar conditions be present, it follows that the children of the patient may also be at risk. As we know, early intervention in most health problems may positively impact the degree of suffering, amount of care, and prospects for a successful outcome.

Fourth, most people, when excited about the successful resolution of their health concerns, often tell others of the success. The family health history form makes the patient aware of other family member

Family Health History

Patient: _____

> Occasionally, a patient's spinal weaknesses and their predisposition to vertebral subluxations are affected by hereditary considerations or their family's lifestyles. Please help us to better understand your family history (and how it may impact your response to chiropractic care) by completing the information below:

Please Check The Appropriate Boxes & Return This Form On Your Next Visit.

CONDITIONS	SPOUSE	FATHER	MOTHER	BROTHER	SISTER	CHILD	CHILD	OTHER
Headaches								
Sinus Problems								
Allergies								
Neck Pain								
Hand/Arm								
Mid-Back								
Chest Pain								
Low Back								
Hip Problems								
Leg Pain								
Nervousness								
Arthritis								
Neuritis								
Throat								
Muscle Pain								
Lungs								
Stomach								
Spinal Curve								
Muscle Spasm								
Female Prob.								
Numbness								
Thyroid Prob.								
Joint Pain								
Eating Disorder								
Other:								

Sample Form: **Family Health History**

who may be suffering. Such awareness often leads the person to help those loved ones by informing them about the benefits they have attained.

Finally, with information regarding the patient's family, you may develop a list of potential patients who can be cultivated as a source of future referrals.

Presentation and Explanation

The procedure for utilizing this form is simple. At the end of the first visit, you should present the form to the patient with the following script:

> **Doctor:** "Mrs. Jones, it will take us a couple of hours to process your films. Later tonight I will sit down and study them and correlate them with your examination findings. Therefore, we have done all that we can today.
>
> "There is one other area that we only briefly touched on, that being the possibility of a genetic weakness that may have contributed to, or allowed your problems to develop.
>
> "Will you complete this form and bring it back tomorrow? It will give us important information on your family history and any genetic overlay that may affect your response to our care.
>
> "I will get your films developed, get my homework done, and be ready for you tomorrow. Do you have any questions?
>
> "Let's go back up to the front desk and make an appointment for tomorrow."

The "Follow-Up" Procedure—Second Visit

The follow-up on this procedure is simple. When the patient returns the form on the following visit, the CA should place the family health history form on the clipboard for the doctor to review prior to the case report. He or she should review the completed form before entering the consultation room. This valuable information will give the doctor a greater degree of insight into the patient's possible rate of recovery, the amount of care required, and the necessity to further investigate the patient's lifestyles and activities.

Then, prior to the case report, the doctor will briefly review the family health history form with the patient and explain any potential for family traits that may be associated with the patient's presenting concerns. Remember, however, this visit is about the patient. Always review and relate these findings to the patient. This is not the time to suggest referrals.

First Reevaluation

Finally, the family health history form should be placed on the patient's clipboard at the patient's first reevaluation. Then, when the doctor re-consults with the patient (and the patient has experienced positive results) you may review the practice mission and offer to consult with any family members who may be experiencing this or similar problems.

> **Doctor:** "Mrs. Jones, you are progressing right on schedule. You are exactly where I hoped you would be at this point. (If true.) Most of your symptoms have been relieved, and we actually have a good start on correcting your spine.
>
> "By the way, on your family health history form that you filled out, you mentioned that your sister has had problems with her spine. Tell me more about her problems." (Let patient relate relative's health concerns) "Since you have already experienced such good results, have you considered having her checked for possible subluxation?"

Or...

> "Since you have experienced such good results, and understand how and why chiropractic works, have you thought about encouraging your sister to have her spine checked for subluxations? If you would like, you can tell Carol where your sister lives, and I can send her some information and recommend a good chiropractor in her area."

If the patient indicates that the family member lives in the area, briefly state the doctor's practice mission of caring for every member of his or her community and, of course, offer to see her sister.

If the patient seems agreeable to bringing in the family member, the rest of the office visit should be completed, and the patient escorted to the front desk for dismissal. Once at the front desk, the doctor should make the following statement to the CA:

> **Doctor:** "Carol...Mrs. Jones is right on schedule and she needs to continue her correction for the next 4 to 6 weeks, but only at three times per

week. Also, would you give her a complimentary consultation and examination card for her sister and try to set aside enough time on her next visit so that I can talk with her too?"

"Mrs. Jones, you are doing great. Let us keep after this until we get it corrected and stabilized. I will see you and your sister on Friday."

Bonus Step 1-6: Make New Patients Happen—the Referral Request Procedure

How many new patients do you want each week? Two? Ten? Twenty-five? It doesn't matter. With the referral request procedure, the choice is yours. This procedure solves two of the biggest problems facing most doctors in today's private practice. One major problem is how to obtain profitable, highly motivated patients who will support the practice's growth objectives. And, how to do it without resorting to costly, and sometimes unprofessional, methods of media advertising and service discounts.

In today's market of managed care and cost containment, the ability to generate a continual source of new patients is vital to every practice's growth and stability. This procedure will allow you to establish a consistent flow of new patients. You will be able to initiate the procedures necessary to help your established patients provide those new patients, virtually at will.

By knowing how to properly ask for new patients, you can use existing relationships to attract high potential, appreciative patients. Most importantly, the procedure allows you to function within a personal comfort zone while attracting only the types of patients who you enjoy having in your practice.

Referral Discipline (Or, how many do you want?)

The referral procedure is simple, the actions easy and professional. They are based on the principles of concern, professionalism, and the desire to serve. But, the commitment to action is fundamental to making this procedure a success. The entire concept of this procedure is useless, unless you and your staff have committed yourselves to taking the few simple steps needed to implement it. Just as in all areas of practice, setting goals is the key to developing the concentration and focus necessary to achieve the desired results. If you can focus on new patients, and concentrate on applying this procedure, then you will be successful in controlling the new patient flow into your practice. Setting the goal and working to achieve it is the real secret of practice growth and new patient acquisition.

Once a specific new patient goal is determined, and these procedures applied, you are finally in control. By becoming aware of the potential referral sources within every current patient and taking time to ask the necessary questions, practice stability and growth is certain.

This procedure is a tool for making new patients happen. Like all tools, it will not benefit its owner unless it is used—and used properly. Study and learn the procedure well. It will clear up the mystery about why some people are so successful at asking for and getting referrals, while most are miserable failures. Practice it often. Make up different scenarios, different patients, and different answers. It works. However, *you* have to work it. If you do, those erratic Yellow Pages calls or random patient referrals will be just "gravy"—or possibly even nuisances.

Key Terms
- Specific feature—A characteristic, trait, or attribute of a person, object, or profession.
- Distinctive benefit—A short, succinct sentence that describes what you do and how it benefits the person using your services.
- Frame of reference—A pattern of thinking that confines one's thought into a specific area or group that is implicated by a specific commonality.
- Tangible accelerator—Something of value that serves as a catalyst in initiating a specific action.
- Suitable prospect—A person who needs your product or services and may be inclined to use them if given the appropriate opportunity.
- Environmental link—A common factor in the lives of two or more people that may precipitate or predispose those persons to similar ailments.

Preliminary Patient Relations

The overwhelming factor in setting the stage for referrals is to develop a warm professional relationship with each patient already in your practice as we described earlier. The patients who will refer others are not necessarily those who have experienced extraordinary results. Strangely, it is not the satisfied patient who routinely tells others about your practice. Instead, it is the patient who is excited and enthusiastic about your practice, your staff, and you—their doctor.

How can we excite our patients? Actually, in this day of high-tech/low-touch, sterile offices, cold ultra-professional specialists, arrogant staffs, and forbidding machines, the patient's need for compassion, concern, and the human touch is greater than ever. People need to be seen as unique individuals with their own special needs, problems, and fears. By simply by "going the extra mile" on a humanistic level, we can reach out to our patients and excite them with our caring and concern. There are literally hundreds of ways to show our patients they are special and that we recognize and appreciate them. There are even more ways to show our patients that we care. We have touched on a few of these methods in the previous sections

In general, you must truly *care* about your patients and your practice. You must serve your patients on a professional yet compassionate plane. Doing so will tell the patients that you, your staff, and your practice are special. When they encounter a practice that is so unusual, so different, most patients will want to tell everyone they know about you and your practice.

How to Ask for Referrals (And get them.)

I believe that most patients want to see their doctor be successful. I also believe that most patients want their doctors to accept them, recognize them as good patients, and appreciate them as someone special. From experience, I know that patients always want to help their friends and family live healthy abundant lives. This is especially true when they have a doctor and staff who are professional, proficient, and have created a warm, caring rapport with the patient. Yet, most doctors have a difficult time asking their patients for referrals because they feel uncomfortable, unprofessional, or just awkward doing so.

"Who do you know who could use my services?"

We have all heard the best way to get referrals is to ask for referrals. Anyone who has tried, however, knows that such action is, by its nature, stressful and somewhat confrontational. The fear of rejection is too great, and the likelihood of a "nobody" answer prevents the average doctor from climbing out onto that limb.

But for most of us, our desire to fulfill our destiny of touching lives and helping people becomes so strong that we decide to go for it. At least once.

We choose a patient with whom we have had a good, long-standing relationship. We know this patient likes us and we like the patient. So on the next visit, quite out of the blue, we "pop" the question: "Mrs. Jones, do you know of anyone who needs my services that you could send to me?"

"I can't think of anyone right now."

Suddenly, we have a brain-dead patient on our hands. The patient's mind just went blank. A glazed stare, shrugged shoulders, and a sense of resentment for being put in such a situation are too typical. The patient feels he or she has been put on the spot and is even somewhat embarrassed. You feel like an unprofessional buffoon and you vow to never make this mistake again.

What went wrong? This was your best patient. If she is unwilling to give you the name of just one of her many friends to refer to you, who will? You should not blame yourself or Mrs. Jones. It was a bad question with even worse timing. In reality, the question was simply too broad and the patient was caught off guard. The problem is compounded by the fact that most of us just know too many people. For Mrs. Jones to single out one or two specific individuals at a moment's notice is difficult.

Joe Girard, author of the book *How to Sell Anything to Anybody*, explains that each of us has a personal sphere of influence of about 250 other people. If you were to multiply the number of patients who are currently your practice by 250, you will quickly see the possibilities of evoking enough new patient referrals that you would never have to advertise. You can easily understand how important knowing how to ask for referrals is to your ability to grow your practice.

However, as with Mrs. Jones, there is a huge downside to each of our patients' having such a huge sphere of influence. That is, if you approach your patient for referrals the wrong way, they will be unable to provide even one name from that vast list. Therefore, it follows that by exploring what we termed their "environmental links" to others, the patient will easily "see" others who might be in need of chiropractic care too.

Step One: Narrow the Person's "Frame of Reference"

A patient's sphere of influence is usually confined to others who have similar activities, lifestyles, and interests. Their friends are typically in the same age group. Their coworkers often perform the same type of job function and have similar physical stresses. Many of the patient's hobbies or sports bring the patient into contact with others who may be subject to activities that produce similar physical consequences.

Instead of asking such an all-encompassing question, it is crucial to anchor the person to a specific pattern of thinking. Such anchoring confines the patient's thought pattern into a specific area that has a common link to the patient's friends and family.

A "frame of reference" directs the patient's thought to a list of only a few possible, yet obvious, referrals. The most successful list is, of course, comprised of those whom the patient has the greatest interaction with and influence over—their inner circle of friends and frequent acquaintances. Such groups may include coworkers, racquetball opponents, golfing buddies, health club members, civic club members, or other social groups. Indeed, any group that the patient is regularly a member of is fertile ground for developing frames of reference.

To be successful, it is important to get to know your patients on a personal level. Their type of work, their social habits, their interests, and their hobbies will all be key leads to prospecting for referrals. Much of the necessary information is gathered via a comprehensive consultation such as we discussed in previous chapters. Every competent doctor needs to explore environmental factors such as hobbies, sports, and requirements of employment in which the patient participates. This gives the doctor a good idea of both the precipitating and complicating factors in the patient's current and long-term health concerns (see "adverse environmental possibilities," consultation item #7 on the patient consultation worksheet).

In addition, it gives great insight into the patient's sphere of influence to be explored later for referral purposes.

Besides developing these insights during the consultation, it is also an important function of the doctor and the rest of the staff to keep their ears open for such clues as they get to know the patient on a more personal level. For instance, if, while booking an appointment, the patient states that Monday is "golf day" or "sewing circle day," the CA should pick up on this and make a note of such activities. Once a specific frame of reference is identified and certain individuals isolated, the doctor can then initiate the referral procedure on this particular frame of reference. Such a process often yields many referrals.

Developing a "Frame of Reference"

By narrowing the number of faces the patient sees when asked about possible referrals, the patient will have a much better likelihood of seeing one friend or relative within that specific "frame" who may display the possible need for chiropractic care. Narrowing the frame of reference not only reduces the vast number of faces that may flash across the patient's mind, but will also *cause* a group of faces to actually materialize.

> **Doctor:** "Mrs. Jones, Carol mentioned that you play cards with the ladies every Tuesday afternoon, is that right?"
>
> **Patient:** "That's right, canasta. Every Tuesday for the past 20 years."
>
> **Doctor:** "Do you always play with the same group of ladies?"
>
> **Patient:** "Yes, there are eight of us. We have been friends since we were girls."

Step 2: Establish an Environmental Link

Exploring the environmental link will help the patient understand how their activities or lifestyle may have played a role in the development of the subluxation complex that brought them to your office. At this point, they probably understand many of the causative factors of their health concerns, but never made the next logical step in recognizing that many of their friends, family, or coworkers are subject to the same activities and possible causative factors. Making such a step in their understanding often empowers the patient to discuss with their friend or family member the possibility of having their spine checked for vertebral subluxation as well.

> **Doctor:** "Mrs. Jones, the problems that brought you to our office are common in women over 60. As far as you know, do any of the ladies you play cards with ever complain about similar problems?"

Patient: "Oh, Sarah Smith has a terrible neck and her asthma caused her to miss last week's game."

Step 3: Patient Empowerment Statement and Question

Once you have identified a specific frame of reference to identify an environmental link, the patient now sees the individual faces of those who may need your services. Now, it is necessary to empower the patient to have the confidence to bring a friend into the office. The patient empowerment statement is a statement used to give the patient the confidence to make the referral.

A typical patient empowerment statement is extremely personal and reflects you and your patient's relationship, your working together to serve the patient and her family and friends.

Your Patient Empowerment Statement

This statement is provided to empower the patient and to give them the confidence that they do have the knowledge and understanding to discuss such concerns with others. At the same time, it subtly lets them know that with this understanding comes the responsibility of sharing their knowledge with others.

Doctor: "I know that you know and understand, Mrs. Jones, how effective chiropractic care can be in cases such as yours and probably Sarah's."

Patient: "I sure do."

Next, you should lead—not push—the patient into making the decision to approach her friend with a referral concept. In any situation, the person who asks the questions controls the conversation. Therefore, rather than ask the patient to refer Sarah to you, you should ask a different type of question. Instead, ask her a question that will successfully lead her to make the decision for herself to refer her friend to you.

Doctor: "Don't you just wish, Mrs. Jones, that everyone understood what we know about how well chiropractic works to allow the body to heal and to sustain itself?" (Wait for the patient to answer in the affirmative.)

"There would sure be a lot less suffering. Do you know if Sarah has ever had her nerve system examined for interference to her lungs?" (Usually, patient will answer in the negative.)

"Since she is your friend, I would like to check her—at my expense. How else could I help you help her?" (If patient does not know how you could help, you may give her a couple of ideas...) "Would you be comfortable bringing her with you the next time you come in? I'm sure she would feel more comfortable with you along."

Or...

"If she would like to give me a call, I would be happy to speak with her by telephone. Would you talk to her?"

Remember, to be most effective and as stress-free as possible, the patient must never feel that your questioning technique is asking her to make a referral. Instead, you are being interested in her and compassionate in your concern for her friends and family.

Also remember that every time during the patient's visit that you open your mouth and talk about yourself, your family, or your interests, you are committing three huge errors in building your practice and doing the patient a grave disservice. First, you are boring your patient. Second, you are missing an opportunity to better educate your patient about chiropractic and the concepts of health and wellness. Third, you are missing a huge opportunity to ask the appropriate questions that will give the patient the opportunity bring their friends and family under chiropractic care.

Step 4: Follow-Through for the Patient

The referral process may be greatly strengthened by your offering to contact the patient personally. Optimally, you, the doctor should call the prospective patient prior to the referring patient's next appointment.

The main point of this call is for you to introduce yourself and explain that you are calling because her friend was concerned about her health. In addition, you should explain how you promised her friend that you would call.

If done correctly, following through for the patient is effective in enrolling the new patient. It may double or triple the results of this procedure. Such an offer should always be presented in a low-key manner. If there is any hesitation by the patient, you should quickly back away from the offer. Such calls are so influential and so successful that you should always make the offer to every patient.

Extend the offer to follow through:

> **Doctor:** "If you like, I would be happy to talk to Sarah. If she would rather just discuss her problem on the phone, I would be happy to do that. So, after you talk to her, would you call Carol and tell her if Sarah would like an appointment or if she would like me to call her?"

Step 5: Offer a "Tangible Accelerator"

The offer of a complimentary examination is, in this case, used as a tangible accelerator. A tangible accelerator is catalyst. It is a physical item designed to hasten the desired actions on the part of the referrer and the prospective patient. Properly used, it is a vital motivator for stimulating the referral. The bestowal of a complimentary consultation and examination card is made to make the referring patient feel special. It should be dated. Dating the offer will give it an air of urgency and value. It will also prevent the referring patient and the prospective new patient from delaying the actions needed to bring the prospective patient into the office.

Offer a tangible accelerator:

> **Doctor:** "I will be happy to see what I can do. Since she is a friend of yours, I'd be happy to talk to her completely at my expense. In fact, if I give you a special complimentary consultation and examination card (or offer a complimentary telephone consultation), can you give it to her also?"

Step 6: Follow-Up Phone Call

Finally, if the patient or the prospective patient would like you to call, you should make a big point of promising Mrs. Jones that you will call her friend in a couple of days (after she's had the chance to give her the card and talk to her). Before she leaves, both you and your staff should sincerely thank the patient for her confidence and for helping her friends.

Within two to three days (giving Mrs. Jones a chance to call her friend), you should call the referring patient. The main point of this call is for you to introduce yourself and explain that you are calling because Mrs. Jones was concerned about her. You should also explain that you promised Mrs. Jones you would call.

> **Doctor:** "Mrs. Smith? This is Dr. Meyer. I am Mrs. Jones' doctor. I don't normally call nonpatients at home, but Mrs. Jones was concerned about you and asked if I thought we could help your with your asthma. I promised her that I would call you and find out. Has she had a chance to mention this to you yet? Is now a convenient time?"

Step 7: Your "Distinctive Benefit" Statement

When the person answers in the affirmative, you should immediately state your distinctive benefit that you probably could help them with their problems, but further information about their case is necessary.

> **Doctor:** "Mrs. Smith, in my office we try to help our patients live as healthy and as abundantly as possible by helping their bodies function as near 100 percent as possible. I have had many patients with symptoms such as yours. Could you tell me a little more about your breathing problems?"

Continue to perform a full consultation at this time. Then when the patient then comes into the office for her first appointment, all the doctor has to do during the consultation is to review what was discussed, and verify the accuracy of his or her notes.

Step 8: Say (and Write) Thank You

If Mrs. Smith makes an appointment, you should immediately call Mrs. Jones and tell her you have spoken with Mrs. Smith and that she will be coming into the office. Then, tell Mrs. Jones how much you appreciate her and value her as a patient. In short, praise her for being such a good patient and such a caring friend. After the new patient's first appointment, a thank-you note is sent immediately to the referring patient.

If Mrs. Smith does not make an appointment, still call Mrs. Jones and tell her you called her friend (as promised). Say that the friend did not make an appointment, but that you left it that she will call if she changes her mind. In addition, a gracious letter should be sent to Mrs. Smith. The gist of the letter is to thank her for her time and to again invite her to call should she have any questions. (Enclose a practice brochure and your curriculum vitae.)

Summary of Entire Script—Putting It Together

Following is a typical script that puts it all together. Visualize this conversation between yourself and one of your current patients. It will give you an idea of just how to use an environmental link to develop a frame of reference, use your distinctive benefits, and identify people who may be suitable prospects:

Frame of Reference

Doctor: "Mrs. Jones, my CA, Carol, mentioned that you play cards with the ladies every Tuesday afternoon, is that right?"

Patient: "Canasta. Every Tuesday for the past 20 years."

Doctor: "Do you always play with the same group of ladies?"

Patient: "Yes, there are eight of us. We have known each other since we were girls."

Environmental Link

Doctor: "Mrs. Jones, the problems that brought you to our office are common in women over 60. As far as you know, do any of the ladies that you play cards with ever complain about similar problems?"

Patient: "Sarah Smith has a terrible neck and her asthma caused her to miss last week's game."

Distinctive Benefit

Doctor: "I know that you know, Mrs. Jones, how effective chiropractic is in cases such as yours and Sarah's. Don't you just wish that everyone understood what we know about how the body works? There would sure be a lot less suffering. Do you know if she has had her nerve system examined for interference?

"Since she is your friend, I would like to offer to check her at my expense. If I would extend to her a complimentary consultation and examination would you bring her in with you on your next visit? I'm sure she would feel more comfortable with you along."

Offer to Follow Through

Doctor: "If you would like, I would be happy to talk to her to see if I could help her before she actually comes into the office. If she would rather just discuss her problem on the phone, I would be happy to do that to. After you talk to her, would you call Carol and tell her if Sarah would like an appointment or if she would like me to call her?"

Tangible Accelerator
Doctor: "I will be happy to see what I can do. In fact, if I give you a special complimentary consultation and examination card (or offer a free Introductory Telephone Consultation), you can give it to her also."
Patient: "Sure, that sounds great."

After the visit, you will then escort Mrs. Jones to the front desk and ask the CA for a complimentary examination card. At this point also, the CA should get Mrs. Smith's phone number. If the patient does not know Mrs. Smith's phone number, the CA should give her the telephone book and help her look it up.

Follow-up Phone Call
Doctor: "Mrs. Smith? This is Dr. Meyer. I am Mrs. Jones' chiropractor. She was concerned about you and I promised her I would call you. Would you like to take a few minutes to discuss your health and explore whether there might be anything we can do to help you?"
Patient: "Sure, I would be happy to."

If "Yes," proceed to a mini-consultation about the problem.
If "No," graciously ask the person if they would like you to call back at a better time. If still "No," respectfully thank them for their time and invite them to call you anytime in the future.

Summary

As mentioned previously, the following is most effective when the referring patient is in a state of unequal exchange with your practice. The perfect time to initiate such a procedure is when the patient first reports improvement, or when you sense that the patient is feeling especially good about you, your staff, and your practice. Remember, it is always service, kindness, concern, and compassion that will lead to a patient who is excited and enthusiastic about you and your staff. Such excitement and enthusiasm make it extremely easy for patients to tell others about you and your practice, thus setting the stage for years of referrals.

Bonus Step 1-7: Remove New Patient Hurdles—the Introductory Telephone Consultation

Program Concept

It is absurd to tell any professional who has ever built or maintained a practice that there is an ongoing need to procure new patients on a consistent and dependable basis. We all know that to create practice growth, as well as maintain an established practice, a flow of new patients is a significant factor. We must still consider every aspect that goes into developing a strong referral practice. In doing so, we must also consider ways to make it easy for both referred and nonreferred prospects to take the first step toward chiropractic care.

The fear of becoming a patient is actually a fear of the unknown. The average prospective patient has many questions, concerns, and trepidations that may delay or prevent them from picking up the telephone and calling for an appointment. If so, it then stands to reason that if we can deal with their concerns without putting them into an unknown or uncomfortable situation, we may open the doors for many more prospective patients to explore you and your practice.

Our experience has led us to consider and experiment with many different ways to allow prospects to investigate our practice. Those that have been the most successful lowered the hurdles for the prospects, making it comfortable for them to make their initial appointment. First, we needed to identify those hurdles. Upon interviewing prospective patients, it became obvious that the average prospective patient had four basic questions (that are only slightly different from those addressed in the case review) that need to be answered:

- What is wrong with me?
- Is it a problem this particular doctor can help me with?
- What needs to be done?
- How much will it cost? (How can I pay for it?)
- Will this doctor and the staff be professional, yet warm and caring individuals?

Most professionals have experimented with various forms of marketing that attempt to answer these questions and ultimately the free-exam concept became popular throughout the professions. The major flaw with the free examination approach is that it still requires the prospect to make the commitment to physically come into the office and encounter you and your staff. Again, apprehension, trepidation, and anxiety always accompany a new patient into any doctor's office.

For many years, we used the complimentary examination concept to lower the initial financial hurdle for referred new patients. But, the complimentary examination seldom produced the high percentage results that we wanted. The reason for this was simple: it required the patient to gather enough courage to call the office, book an appointment, and physically come to the office and face their anxieties and apprehensions.

We must remember that at this point we are still dealing with prospective patients who are hesitant to physically come into the office because of their fear of the unknown. For this reason, we must find a way to answer questions and ease concerns without placing them in a situation where they may feel trapped or at a psychological disadvantage.

These feelings can be greatly reduced simply by allowing the patient to get to know you prior to coming into the office for the first time. The best way to accomplish this is to make it possible for the prospective patient to speak to you without the face-to-face confrontation they may be knowingly or unknowingly trying to avoid.

It became our goal to develop a way for a prospective new patient to make an appointment and physically come into the office without any of the previous fears or concerns. The result was a marketing concept known as the Introductory Telephone Consultation.

Built on the Referral Request Procedure

In every instance, the referral request procedure can be greatly enhanced by offering the referring patient the opportunity to extend the Introductory Telephone Consultation as a tangible accelerator. Such a procedure actually sets the stage for the patient to develop a frame of reference as well as become motivated to take the steps necessary to follow through on the actual referral.

We have found that utilizing a tangible accelerator (something of value that serves as a catalyst in initiating a specific action) is very effective. In this case, the offer of your availability to talk to patients before they ever come into the office is used as an effective tangible accelerator. In many instances, the tandem use of an Introductory Telephone Consultation and a complimentary consultation and examination certificate makes the ultimate conversion of the patient much easier.

Implementation Procedures

The Introductory Telephone Consultation procedure is effective in three situations:

1. When you are prospecting for new patients by using the referral request procedure.
2. When an established patient brings to your attention the existence of someone they have been trying to refer but who is reluctant.
3. When a prospective new patient calls the office with questions or concerns that the CA cannot answer.

The Referral Request Procedure

The referral request procedure is very effective in narrowing the patient's frame of reference, establishing an environmental link, and using your distinctive benefit to qualify prospective referrals. You can then greatly increase the referring patient's effectiveness by offering the Introductory Telephone Consultation to the patient.

> **Doctor:** "Mrs. Jones, I would be happy to see what I can do for your friend. And, since she is a friend of yours, I'd be happy to talk with her by phone first, or I can offer her a complimentary examination."

Or...

> "If I give you a special complimentary consultation and examination card (or offer a complimentary telephone consultation), will you give it to her?"

If the patient agrees, you should leave the subject immediately and continue with the patient's visit. At the completion of the visit, escort the patient to the front desk and ask the CA to complete the procedure:

> **Doctor:** "Carol, Mrs. Jones has a friend we may be able to help. Would you give her a complimentary consultation and examination certificate and explain the Introductory Telephone Consultation to her?

"Thank you, Mrs. Jones. I'll see you on Friday, I hope we can get your friend in and help her too."

Bonus Step 1-8: Stay Alert for the Reluctant Referral

Very often, a patient will ask you (or staff members) about certain conditions and wonder if chiropractic can benefit such a condition. In such an instance, you and your staff should be alert to the fact that patients seldom make up conditions simply to quiz the doctor. They ask for a reason, and that reason is usually a friend, coworker, or family member with just such a problem.

An alert doctor will never miss this opportunity, but will seize this situation in a caring, compassionate, professional way to explore why this particular question was asked. After a brief discussion of the problem or condition, you should turn the conversation to the prospective patient.

Doctor: "Mrs. Jones, is there a reason you've asked about this?"

Patient: "Yes, the man who works next to me at the office is having this type of problem and we are all worried about him."

Doctor: "Have you talked with him about what you know about chiropractic? And encouraged him to be checked for vertebral subluxation and especially nerve interference?

"If he is a little reluctant, I would be happy to talk to him by phone and answer any questions he may have. You know, my mission is to (state your practice mission), and I would be happy to do whatever is necessary to see if chiropractic might help him. Do you think if I talked to him I might be able to answer his concerns?"

Patient: "I am sure you could. Let me talk to him tomorrow at work…"

Doctor: "That would be fine. When you leave, I will have Carol give you an Introductory Telephone Consultation brochure and a certificate for a complimentary consultation and examination. Please give them to him and then let Carol know if he would like me to phone him."

♦ Generate New Patient Referrals ♦

If patient agrees, leave the subject immediately, and at the completion of the visit, escort the patient to the front desk and ask the CA to complete the procedure:

> **Doctor:** "Carol, Mrs. Jones has a friend we may be able to help. Would you give her a complimentary consultation and examination certificate, and explain the Introductory Telephone Consultation program to her?
>
> "Thank you, Mrs. Jones. I'll see you on Friday; I hope we can get your friend in and help him too."

At this point, the CA should first explain the Introductory Telephone Consultation brochure to the patient and make certain that she understands it, and then complete and give the complimentary consultation and examination certificate to the referrer. Once that is completed, he or she should then enter the names of the referrer and the prospective patient along with all pertinent information in the complimentary consultation and examination log book.

Bonus Step 1-9: Turn Inquiries into Patients—the Prospective Patient Phone Call

Our staff used to hate the prospective patient who would call with what seemed to be a list of stupid questions. "What does a chiropractor do?" "How much is the first visit?" "Do I need x-rays?" "Can chiropractic help hemorrhoids?" And on and on. The staff wanted to be helpful, they wanted to be honest, and they even wanted to book that caller as a new patient. Unfortunately, all too often they succeeded at none of these.

Finally, I realized the reason they hated these calls is because I never gave them answers to these questions. They simply could not know the answers. They did not know what x-rays would be indicated. They had no idea what level of exam would need to be performed. And, they certainly did not know if the patient was subluxated and if chiropractic could help. Once we realized that the same questions were being asked over and over, we knew that if we could just provide effective answers these calls would not be quite so frustrating. With a little work and

Sample Form: **Prospective Patient Log**

◆ Generate New Patient Referrals ◆

planning, we soon had the proper scripts and such calls actually became a game the staff looked forward to.

So what are some of these questions, and how should they be answered? One of the most difficult, yet most common, calls for your front desk staff to answer is the prospective patient who is inquiring as to various clinical indications, protocols, and fees associated with the first visit. This is difficult because neither you nor your CA have any way of telling what level examination will be required.

As soon as the CA realizes the prospective patient has questions that cannot be answered, he or she should immediately offer the caller the opportunity of scheduling an Introductory Telephone Consultation with the doctor.

> **CA:** "We have a special service for prospective patients who have just such questions. If you wish, the doctor would be happy call you this afternoon. At that time (he or she) can discuss your situation, your health history, and whether you may be a good prospect for chiropractic care. There is no cost or obligation, and if the doctor can help you, (he or she) can better answer your questions about fees at that time. If (he or she) feels that (he or she) cannot help you, (he or she) will steer you in the right direction. How does that sound?
>
> "May I have your name, phone number (etc.)?
>
> "The doctor will be free this evening about 6:00...would it be convenient for him to call you then?"

It is vital that the CA set a specific time and place for you to call the patient so you do not waste your time and the patient does not become frustrated waiting for your call.

Preparation by the staff and the doctor are critical for the success of this phone call. After the CA has gathered the information needed for you to call the prospective patient, he or she should begin to assemble a new patient folder for the doctor's use during the actual call. Such a folder must include:

◆ All information gathered about the patient by the CA (brief nature of problem, referring patient, etc.)

◆ A new patient consultation worksheet

◆ A list of fees for new patient services for you to refer to if necessary

♦ A list of times available for a possible new patient appointment on the following day

To gain a true understanding of the patient, it is important that the doctor allow the patient to do most of the talking during the telephone interview. Focus the conversation on the patient and their concerns. Try to put yourself in the patient's place. The patient is probably looking for a doctor who understands them and is willing to listen. Therefore, this is an excellent time to begin the process of filling out the patient's consultation worksheet. In fact, as the consultation progresses be sure to paraphrase the patient's information back to them to prove you are listening and understand their problems and their concerns.

Then, when completed you can use a variation of the second transition statement to inform the patient of what you would recommend as you would a patient who is actually sitting in the consultation room.

Doctor: "Mrs. Jones, is there anything I should have asked or you would like to know that we did not cover before we go on?

"If not, our next step is try to discover the true underlying cause of your complaints. To do this, we should examine your entire spine and nerve system. Also, we need to see if there are any other problems that may be developing as a result of: (list any previous falls, accidents, or injuries that were discussed during the consultation).

"If I can find the cause of your problem and I feel I can help you, I will. But, if not, I will tell you that right away and I will help you to find someone who might.

"Before I called this evening, Carol mentioned we had an opening for a new patient exam at 10:00 A.M. and 2:00 P.M. tomorrow. Would you like to reserve one of those times?"

In most cases, the patient will have already accepted you and have decided to make an appointment. If he or she does not, or if the appointment is set for sometime later than a day or two, a follow-up letter thanking the patient for her time and expressing your pleasure at being able to talk with him or her will be appreciated and well accepted. Never badger or even encourage the patient to make an appointment past the initial offering of the two times stated earlier. If the patient hesitates to schedule an appointment, always leave the door open; be gracious, warm, and professional.

Also remember, that now is not the time to chiropractically enlighten the patient or even to describe in detail what you think she might need beyond the initial examination.

Summary

The Introductory Telephone Consultation procedure has several benefits that are readily apparent. First, this procedure quickly gets the CA "off the hook" and out of a time-consuming and stressful situation when a caller has questions. Second, this procedure stops the caller from further "shopping." This procedure will also effectively keep the caller from booking an appointment in another office, knowing that you will be calling her back. Third, and most importantly, it allows you to establish an immediate bond with the patient before they ever come into the office.

Although many doctors will tell you that the referred patient makes the best patient, we have found that this procedure actually makes both the referred and unreferred patient a better patient by establishing a strong bond before they ever enter the office.

Bonus Step 1-10: Ask Subliminally—Use Complimentary Consultation and Exam Certificates

Another easy way to stimulate your patients to refer others is to have an ample supply of complimentary consultation and examination certificates available and visible in your adjusting rooms. These cards should be placed throughout the office where the patients, you, and your staff will see them. Because we want these to be special and of value they should not be left in a place where they will actually be picked up by the patients. Instead, they should be placed strategically throughout the office where the patient will see them, but the doctor must endorse and present them.

We have found that these certificates will stimulate referrals merely by their presence. They subliminally announce to the patient that the practice is accepting new patients and their doctor is willing to "go the extra mile" for patients and their possible referrals.

Whenever a patient asks about the cards or begins to discuss a possible referral, you should perform a brief in absentia consultation. Here you should briefly ask all the pertinent questions and gather the specific details about the patient that show the referring patient that you have a real interest in helping their friend or relative.

Following that, you must offer to consult and examine the patient. Here, the complimentary consultation and examination certificate will again become the tangible accelerator. After presenting the certificate to the patient, you should write the name of the prospective patient on a daily list to be given to the CA. Then, when the prospective patient calls for an appointment, the CA will know how to properly orient this patient as to what will occur on their complimentary visit.

The biggest problem that may arise with the referral certificate is that the new patient may not know what is included, or where the "complimentary" portion of the visit ends and the "payment" portion begins. It is important that this be made clear to the patient up front so that there are no misunderstandings, surprises for the patient, or appearances of "bait and switch" tactics.

This can be easily taken care of when the prospective patient calls for an appointment. If the caller mentions that they possess a complimentary consultation and examination certificate, or when the CA notices their name is on the list of referral certificates the doctor has given to patients, the CA can proceed with the following advisory script:

Referral Certificate
Complimentary New Patient Consultation & Examination

Courtesy Of
DR. MICHAEL S. MEYER

Special Recipient

Referring Patient | Valid Until

Includes:
Complete Case Consultation, Health History & Analytical Procedures Necessary To Determine If Chiropractic Care Might Enhance The Health & Well-Being Of The Recipient.
*Does not include possible x-rays or clinical care.

Sample Form: **Referral Certificate**

CA: "Mrs. Jones, let me give you an idea of what to expect when you come in Monday for your complimentary consultation with the doctor and your examination.

"First, we will gather all the necessary information about your health and your health history. There will be a few brief forms to fill out. The doctor will spend some time with you discussing your health history and your present concerns. Then, if you wish the doctor will perform an examination of your spine and nerve system. It is thorough and it normally would cost $ (insert number). But, in your case, thanks to (name of referrer) there will be no cost at all.

"When we finish, the doctor will explain what your examination shows. He will also advise you whether or not yours may be a chiropractic case. If so, and you want to begin care, we will schedule you for a more in-depth exam and, if necessary, x-rays, the next day. If you don't, that's okay too. There is absolutely no cost or obligation on your part. Do you have any questions? Good, do you know where our office is located? I'll look forward to seeing you Monday at 10:30. Thank you, Mrs. Jones."

Summary

If you are serious about stimulating high-quality, patient-referred new patients, you must set goals for (and keep track of) the number of referral certificates you present to patients in any given day. Being conscious of the many possibilities for stimulating patient referrals during the day is the best way to fill your ideal practice with new patients.

Using the techniques described in this chapter will give you a controllable and reliable source of high quality new patients. These techniques are neither difficult nor confrontational. In fact, they are just the opposite. You simply have to have your mind in the right place every minute that you interact with every patient. Remember, most patients have the ability and, if treated properly, the desire to bring new patients into your office by the bucketfuls. But, they need help. They need guidance. And most of all, they need to know you have room for and a desire to serve more patients.

If you do not stimulate and encourage new patient referrals, who will?

Key Points

- The procurement of new patients is not a magical, mystical procedure, but merely the end result of proper office procedures, providing positive clinical results, and caring for your patients as you would want your own family cared for.

  The number of referred new patients who come into the practice is the best indication of the doctor's ability to interact properly with the patient, the staff's efficiency, and sound office procedures.

- You must create an environment where the patient feels "obliged" to help you build your practice.

- A healthcare class is the single greatest practice builder known to the chiropractic profession.

- We all know that to create practice growth, as well as maintain an established practice, a flow of new patients is a significant factor.

- The information from the family health history form may have a significant impact on the type of care rendered, as well as the clinical management of the case.

- Frequently, a patient will ask you (or staff members) about certain conditions and wonder if chiropractic can benefit such a condition. An alert doctor never misses this opportunity to seize this situation in a caring compassionate, professional way to explore why this particular question was asked.

- Being conscious of the many possibilities for stimulating patient referrals during the day is the best way to fill your ideal practice with new patients.

Bonus Solution 2

Make Success Personal

As we discussed in the early chapters of this book, success can only come from a solid foundation based on your personal and chiropractic values. This foundation consists primarily of the policies and systems you ultimately develop to reflect your personality and the type of practice you desire. Following are a few of the initial preparations you may want to consider as you begin to climb the stairway to success. As you will soon see, these considerations are important for both your life and your practice. Each will make you a stronger person who is able to make appropriate decisions, communicate your thoughts and concerns, and ultimately, to find the naturally right solutions to the practice of your dreams.

Bonus Step 2-1: Learn to Communicate, Learn to Influence

The most important skill in assuring your success is the ability to communicate and positively influence others on an individual level and, yes, even to speak in public. We have all heard the quote from Andrew Carnegie that more people are afraid of speaking in public than of dying. However, from talking to loan officers at banks and county rezoning boards, to interacting with the first new patient that comes into your office, to giving patient lectures or making presentations before community groups, you must be able to speak well and communicate effectively. Therefore, if you are afraid and do not learn to communicate one-on-one and speak in public, your practice will most assuredly suffer.

I am certain that your new vision of your practice involves how your practice will impact the health and lives of your patients and your community. If so, you must have the ability to communicate it distinctly and succinctly. Without the ability to communicate your vision it will never be realized.

We all remember how Lee Iacocca communicated his vision for the Chrysler Corporation to Congress in order to attain government loans to bail out the languishing automaker. It was that same ability to communicate that helped him to go before the American public in a series of advertisements and "sell" that same vision and his cars to the country. It was not only Lee Iacocca's vision of his company's future that saved Chrysler, but also his ability to communicate that vision. Without Iacocca's ability to communicate his vision, where do you think Chrysler would be today? Likewise, if you do not have the ability to communicate your vision of a desired future state to your patients, where will your practice be tomorrow?

If you have any doubts as to your ability to speak in public, you should take immediate steps to brush up on your communication skills. Whether you take a course in public speaking at a local community college or join Toastmasters, the time taken and the effort made to learn to speak in public will pay off in the months and years to come. Besides speaking in public, such training will help you refine your ideas and delivery in one-on-one situations, making you a better overall communicator. Remember that the ability to communicate is the ability to influence others to make the necessary decisions to do what is best for them, and ultimately for you and your practice.

The other half of communicating is listening. Listening is the ability to concentrate on the spoken word of another person in order to get their meaning. Good listening skills will give you information and clues on how you can give others what they want, understand their fears, and have more satisfying interactions with others. Listening demands effort, intellectual as well as emotional. Listening is a learned skill also, but it is more a skill of concentration and self-discipline.

Bonus Step 2-2: Become Overwhelmingly Confident—in Your Technique and in Yourself

Another step toward success is to become an expert in your core chiropractic technique. Your success in managing patients for their own good, will be based entirely on both your clinical and interpersonal skills. But to a great extent, these skills will be wasted if there is a low degree of confidence and certainty in those skills. Whether you are recently out of school or have been in practice for 50 years, you must concentrate on becoming highly proficient and confident in the technique you choose to use. Fortunately, confidence comes with proficiency.

In addition to your clinical practice, I suggest you attend as many seminars in your chosen technique as you can find time for and afford. If you are a rookie or a veteran in practice, try to visit other practices where you may learn new clinical applications or practical patient management tips that will make you more effective and confident in your professional and technical ability. (Even if you learn nothing new, and only realize that your technical abilities are superior to others, this knowledge, if humbly applied, will make you a more confident practitioner.) If you are still a student, you might seek out internships and preceptorships with doctors who are known for their expertise in your chosen technique or desired type of practice. In short, learn all you can so that when the real test of your skills and knowledge comes, you will be confident, competent, and ready. The greatest asset a healer has is the self-confidence and clinical sureness needed to instill that same confidence in others.

Bonus Step 2-3: Never "Settle"—Purposefully Build Your Perfect Practice and Life

If you have been in practice for some time, now is a good time to stop and ask yourself this important question: "Is my current practice any resemblance of the practice that I envisioned as an idealistic student, or even just a few pages back in this book?" If you have completed the exercise in the introduction of the book and actually visualized your ideal practice, you probably have answered this question already. So now I am asking you...*Is your practice a reflection of your earlier vision of what your practice would become?* And, much more importantly...*Are your core personal and chiropractic values reflected in the way you are practicing?* If the answer to either is "no," and you do not currently have the practice you once dreamed of, my last question to you is...*WHY? Why have you failed to build your ideal practice?*

It is most likely that, in the early days of your practice, you settled for a practice that just "happened." Or, possibly you compromised your chiropractic values. Did you, by any chance, change your rules and begin to play by those of some insurance company? (Or worse...Medicare?) Or, were you simply not able to enact the policies, procedures, or systems that would have given birth to the practice of your dreams. These questions are important and deserve careful consideration—even some serious soul-searching. The answers to these questions will give you insight as to why your practice is less fulfilling and more stressful than it should be.

If the practice you envisioned does not resemble your current practice, I guarantee you are not nearly as successful as you could be. You most likely have developed a practice that has turned into a daily grind that is draining your energy and enthusiasm. If so, with the ideas and systems presented in this book, you can begin to build the practice you want. You can design the practice you will look forward to returning to every morning for the rest of your life...the practice that will refresh your spirit, nourish your soul, and renew your enthusiasm.

Bonus Step 2-4: Never "Settle"— Be Happy Where You Are, or Move

After you have figured out what technique you will become proficient in and the type of practice you wish to build, you next need to determine whether or not you have established your practice in the right location. The old cliché is to merely practice in a location where you want to live. Unfortunately, many start practicing in an area that looks like fertile soil, only to discover later it is not where they want to live and raise their family. On the other hand, the "place you want to live" may not be able to sustain the type of practice you wish to build. Therefore, it is important you make this decision carefully and with great thought…it will affect your quality of life for as long as you live and practice in that location.

To be successful and ultimately happy in the long term, you must give serious thought as to where you wish to live the rest of your personal and professional life. It has been proven throughout our history that a chiropractic practice can be successful anywhere people live. For the most part, your task is merely to decide where you want to be successful. Do you enjoy cold, moderate, or warm climates? Metropolitan or rural settings? Big city or small town? Mountains or oceans? Desert or forest? Do you want to live near your hometown and extended family? Where you grew up, or far away?

It is vital that you strive to establish your practice in an area that will suit your lifestyle and where you will be happiest. The only exception may be that you need to balance the area where you wish to live and practice with the type of practice you wish to have. For example, if you wish to build a sports-injury practice you may find it necessary to locate near a large university or a city with professional or semi-professional sports teams. In other words, make sure that a sufficient population exists to support your desired type of practice.

If you are currently in practice, you may understand this point even more acutely now than when you established your practice. Are you happy in your current location or have you "settled" for the area because that just happens to be where your practice is? If you are not really satisfied, truly happy, I suggest you investigate selling your practice and relocating to the place you really want to live the rest of your life. Remember that life is too short to "settle."

On the other hand, if you are beginning a new practice, think seriously about your location preferences. Do it as "right" as possible from the beginning. If you are about to redesign and rebuild an existing practice, think about your location or relocation preferences. Then, once the decision has been made as to where you wish to practice, you must secure the information needed to acquire licensure in that state. Also, do not forget to investigate the scope of practice laws, and the chiropolitical environment in the state. Make sure everything is congruent with the type of practice you wish to establish. If you are currently a senior student, it is important that you have narrowed the area where you want to practice at least six to eight months before graduation. Obtaining multiple licenses in a given region of the country may serve you well if you find an opportunity in a neighboring state or wish to relocate later. Most colleges and the Internet can provide the necessary information on when state licensure examinations will be held, where the testing and interview will be, what will be required and tested, and what fees are involved.

Bonus Step 2-5: Find a Mentor— Form a "Master-Mind Alliance"

Whether you are new in practice or a veteran, everyone needs a mentor or at least another like-minded friend to form a "master-mind alliance" with. Besides getting to know the successful doctors in the area where you are interested in practicing, it is also a tremendous advantage to find a mentor who will help and guide you to success. If you are new in practice, you may easily develop a mentoring relationship with one of the doctors you have taken to lunch, but mentors may be found anywhere. It is vital you choose your mentors wisely. They provide a great influence on your life and practice.

Undoubtedly, a mentor or friend will be your greatest asset in your ultimate success. Try to find someone you admire, and who is generally admired by the profession for either his or her personal and professional abilities. A mentor should be someone who is both successful and who holds the same values as you. Look for someone who has the knowledge you need, then work to develop a mutually rewarding relationship based on friendship and service. The good news is that every successful chiropractor I have ever met wants to be a mentor and is more than willing to share their knowledge of chiropractic and practice to advance the profession they love. Many even seek out students.

If you are currently a student, the best way to find a mentor is through an internship or preceptorship while still in college. If such a program is not available, you may simply offer to assist a local doctor in her or his office without pay. By offering to develop and analyze films, change headrest paper, assist with examinations, or even clean the office, you will soon become immersed in the aura of chiropractic and the success that permeates the successful practice. Be careful, however, to choose your chiropractic friends and mentors carefully. Avoid those who are negative or sarcastic, or who do not share your chiropractic principles and life values. You may fall prey to these negative attributes just as you may grow with those you wish to develop or reinforce.

If you are currently in practice, you know we all have a tendency to retreat professionally into the cocoons of our offices and individual lives. This is one of the gravest mistakes a chiropractor can make. We need to be emotionally and intellectually stimulated on a regular basis. I strongly suggest that you begin immediately to form a master-mind alliance with other successful chiropractors and other inspirational individuals in your area. As with your "dream team" staff, the benefit of engaging the forces of synergy is that they powerfully amplify the positive results attained by interacting with positive, motivating people.

Whether you are new in practice or a veteran, everyone needs a mentor or at least a confidant to form a master-mind alliance with. That is why you must continually stimulate your thinking process. Even if you are in your final year of chiropractic college, it is never too early or too late to obtain the success and business knowledge that may not have been taught in college—at least not on a practical level. Such knowledge of basic practice success principles and practice procedures will be vital to building and sustaining a successful practice. By learning how to handle real patients, manage a real office, file insurance, and deal with managed-care systems, you can—you must—prepare yourself to succeed. If a mentor on a business level cannot be found, a new doctor, especially, must attend various business management and insurance seminars and maybe even hire a good consultant.

Bonus Step 2-6: Never Stop Learning— Take Business and Success Seminars

One of the biggest mistakes I see doctors make is to get out of school, go into practice, and stop learning. Since you are reading this book, it is obvious that you do not fall into this group. But next time you are at a re-licensure seminar, look around the room. Notice those doctors who are simply putting in their "butt" time. They are so easy to spot. These are the doctors who may sleep during the presentation, reading a book, or playing with their handheld computer game with the sound turned off. Then, if you have the opportunity, look at their practices. I predict these are the same doctors whose practices are not doing so well. These doctors have lost interest. They have not kept up with the exciting developments in our profession. They are not "learners." My grandmother, who lived to be a sharp 99 years young, once told me that it is more important to be "interested" than to be "interesting." The secret to longevity and success in life, as well as practice, is to remain interested and to continue to learn.

Many good seminars are being taught where you can learn how to conduct your practice, handle insurance, deal with managed care, and even market your practice. Although seminars and consultants may appear expensive, they may be better investments than even your adjusting table. Often the initial fees for a top-notch consultant are reduced for first-year practitioners. Just as often, these business seminars or consultancy programs can be financed in your initial startup loan. Don't reinvent the wheel. Get the information you need to make all the right decisions from the day you graduate.

Programs such as those delivered under the auspices of various colleges and state associations are usually the best places to start. Look at the continuing education offered in this field at local colleges and universities.

Conclusion

As we discussed earlier, your degree of personal success is intimately linked to your degree of satisfaction and sense of fulfillment your practice provides. You will note that nowhere above was it mentioned that success is linked to money. As Dr. James Parker used to teach, "Money is merely the by-product of services rendered." In other words, render the services that you have confidence and a strong belief in, and you will naturally attract an abundance of patients and success. Be concerned with building a high-quality, proactive practice, a practice that anticipates potential factors that will cause it to drift off course, and a practice based on your values, your desires, and your principles...the money will follow. To remain true to your dreams and personal values is much more important than money or the trappings of success. The truly successful practice can be built only around these central concepts.

◆ Make Success Personal ◆

Key Points

- If you have any doubts as to your ability to speak in public, take immediate steps to brush up on your communication skills.
- Your success in managing patients on a clinical level will be based entirely on your clinical skills and your degree of confidence and certainty in those skills.
- If the practice you envisioned does not resemble your current practice, then you are not nearly as successful as you could be.
- It is vital that you strive to establish your practice in an area that will suit your lifestyle and where you will be happiest.
- Whether you have been established for some time or are in your senior year of chiropractic college, it is always good to develop personal and professional relationships in the area where you practice or intend to practice.
- Whether you are new in practice or a veteran, everyone needs a mentor or at least another like-minded friend to form a mastermind alliance with.
- Don't reinvent the wheel. Get the information you need to make all the right decisions from the day you graduate. Whether from other chiropractors, seminars, or consultants, the money spent will be an investment that is likely to return manyfold throughout the years to come.

Bonus Solution 3

Quantify Your Achievements, Then Celebrate

Keeping track of how your practice is doing on a week-to-week, month-by-month, and annual basis is critical in determining whether the principles, policies, and activities you have established are working the way you believe they are. Without practice statistics, it is hard to tell where you are or where you are going.

As your practice rapidly evolves into the practice that is, by your terms, successful, you will find you must continue to make ongoing improvements in your office, technique, staff, and policies and procedures. This is only natural and essential for growth.

It is just as important to understand that "changes" that aren't actually "improvements" will lead you nowhere, unless you quantify that they work. Without measuring every aspect of your practice on a regular basis, you are a ship in the dark, steaming ahead with no maps, lights, or compass. You simply cannot know whether you are moving toward your objective, away from it, going in circles, or heading straight for the rocky shores of disaster.

For example, suppose you begin a new patient education lecture designed to attract new patients and to increase your patient retention. But, even with the noblest intentions, what if you did everything wrong? Perhaps you were heavy-handed in getting patients to attend this lecture and your patients came to resent the policies you instituted to get them there. Possibly you presented a poorly designed program that reflected badly on you and your practice. What if your delivery and materials were uninspiring? Maybe the patients who did attend this lecture were so turned off by the whole experience they never gave you another referral and many quit coming altogether. How long would you continue this program?

Unless you were able to quantify the effects of this procedure you have no way of telling if your efforts were steering you toward your goals or taking you further away from them. What if you were so motivated and so determined, that you stubbornly continued this program until your entire practice actually disappeared? Sadly, not only would you not know what happened to your practice, but also without quantifying your procedures, you would never have seen it coming. Keeping basic week-to-week, month-to-month statistical comparisons is imperative. It is never too early or too late in practice to begin doing so.

To begin, office statistics are easy and fun to keep. They may be done in a ledger book, on customized sheets, or by computer. (There are many spreadsheet programs available that can automatically calculate and help you analyze your practice.) If you have purchased a computer in the last few years, it probably already has Microsoft Works or Microsoft Excel installed. These programs are easy to learn and will give you everything you need to set up your spreadsheets and track your practice.

Bonus Step 3-1: See the Entire Picture— Statistical Categories

There are eleven basic statistical categories needed to properly track and manage your practice. Monitoring each category will give you a comprehensive view of every aspect of your practice. Therefore, it is advisable to track the numbers in each of the following categories on a weekly basis:

◆ Quantify Your Achievements, Then Celebrate ◆

Practice Statistics Worksheet

MONTH OF:

Comments:

Week 1	MON	TUE	WED	THU	FRI	SAT	TOTAL
Sched. Patients							
Kept Apts.							
Missed Apts.							
Walk-Ins							
New Patients							
Services							
Collections							

Week 2	MON	TUE	WED	THU	FRI	SAT	TOTAL
Sched. Patients							
Kept Apts.							
Missed Apts.							
Walk-Ins							
New Patients							
Services							
Collections							

Week 3	MON	TUE	WED	THU	FRI	SAT	TOTAL
Sched. Patients							
Kept Apts.							
Missed Apts.							
Walk-Ins							
New Patients							
Services							
Collections							

Totals

Week 4	MON	TUE	WED	THU	FRI	SAT	TOTAL
Sched. Patients							
Kept Apts.							
Missed Apts.							
Walk-Ins							
New Patients							
Services							
Collections							

Patient Visit Average | Collection Percentage | Missed Apt. Percentage | Loss Income From MA's | Referral Percentage | Avg. Income Per Visit | Avg. Income Per Case

Week 5	MON	TUE	WED	THU	FRI	SAT	TOTAL
Sched. Patients							
Kept Apts.							
Missed Apts.							
Walk-Ins							
New Patients							
Services							
Collections							

Sched. Patients | Kept Apts. | Missed Apts. | New Patients | Referrals | Services | Collections

Sample Form: **Statistics Worksheet**

1. *Services*—Services are the total dollar amount of all charges made to all patients for the services rendered in your office. This is the actual yardstick that measures the overall volume of business done based on the total dollar amount of your rendered services. This category includes both new and established patients.
2. *Collections*—Collections are the actual number of dollars brought into the office through the efforts of the front desk and the insurance/billing department.
3. *Scheduled Patients*—Scheduled patients are the total number of patients who have been given an appointment time written in the appointment book. Patients who appropriately cancel or reschedule their appointments are not counted as scheduled appointments.
4. *Patient Visits*—Patient visits are the total number of visits made by all patients (except new first-visit patients). This category includes multiple visits by a patient on the same day, as well as reactivated patients.
5. *New Patients*—New patients refer to the initial visit made by a patient. A new patient is someone who has never been seen in your office before.
6. *Reevaluations*—Reevaluations are procedures that are utilized to measure and monitor a patient's progress while under active care. The reevaluation procedure is a critical element in producing patient compliance of the multiple appointment programs, as well as for justification of care.
7. *Case Management Plan*—This is the tangible execution of the case plan. It is made up of actual appointments for care and reevaluation.
8. *Reactivated (Inactive) Patients*—A reactivated patient refers to the initial visit of a patient who is an established patient, but has not been seen in the office for a predetermined period (usually 9 to 12 months). Most commonly, this visit includes a consultation update, new exam and x-rays, and certainly a new diagnosis.

9. *Missed (Failed) Appointment*—A missed appointment occurs when a patient fails to appear for a scheduled appointment without adequate notice. Patients who show up for their appointment, but are more that 15 minutes late are considered missed and rescheduled.
10. *Rescheduled Missed Appointments*—A rescheduled missed appointment refers to the failed appointments that have been rescheduled either by the action of the patient or the staff.
11. *Case Management Plan Dropouts*—This statistic represents the number of patients who discontinue their multiple appointment programs prematurely.

Bonus Step 3-2: Running the Numbers— Quantitative and Objective Insights

Now that you understand the previous numbers, you can put them to work to track where your practice is doing well, and where you may be drifting off course. Using these numbers to give you better insight into your practice trends and the effects of any policy or procedural alterations is the next step quantitatively and objectively understanding your practice. I have found it beneficial to assign the task of counting and recording the actual numbers to a trusted CA. However, I prefer to make these important computation myself.

Although it is important to track, even graph the statistical categories, it is vital that the same is done with the computations so that you can watch and anticipate trends. It's usually fun, eye-opening, and makes one ponder the messages these numbers are projecting. Along with the recording of the "stats and comps" on a month-by-month, year-by-year basis, it is helpful to make specific notations as to events, procedural and policy changes, or any other factor that will influence these numbers. Only by tying your statistics to events, can you tell if your improvements are really improvements.

An example of tying your statistics to specific practice events may be the institution of a program to bring the new patient's spouse to the initial case review whenever possible. Desiring to do so, the doctor and staff may embark on a program to invite the spouse, to book the case review at a time when the spouse can attend, and to call the evening prior to the review and remind the spouse, maybe even require the spouse's attendance.

By watching your practice statistics both before and after the initiation of this effort, you can soon tell if it is having the desired effects on your practice. If it is, you might expect to see your new patient volume increase as more spouses decide to come under care, and you may see more children come into the practice as mothers and fathers become knowledgeable of the benefits of chiropractic care in their children's development. You may even notice that the average visits per patient (PVA) increases due to better follow-through by your patients because of spouse encouragement.

Having an established baseline of all of these statistics prior to initiating any new policies or procedures, then monitoring them will allow you to objectively determine if your new tactics are having desired, or even undesirable, effects on your practice.

Likewise, keeping track of other events such as inclement weather, vacations, new staff, or any other happenings that might affect your practice statistics will give you both current and historical insights into the growth of your practice.

Patient Visit Average

The patient visit average is possibly the most important and telling formula of all. It shows the average number of visits each new patient will ultimately represent in an office. It is a good indicator of patient longevity, plus your ability to manage patients past initial relief care and into corrective, stabilization, and wellness care.

$$\textit{Formula: Patient Visit Average} = \frac{\text{\# of Patient Visits}}{\text{\# of New Patients}}$$

A low patient visit average usually represent high attrition rates caused by patients who are prematurely dropping out of care. If you have patients who do not stay under care and progress through the clinical objectives of condition-based care, or who do not accept the concept of health and development care, this number will be low. There is no limit as to how high a PVA may be in an established practice. I have seen practices with PVAs in the hundreds. In a typical established practice that is doing well and accepting a good number of new patients, the average PVA seems to be around 30. Remember that one side of the PVA equation is "new patients." Therefore, if you have a month where new patients are high, your PVA will drop. On the other hand, if you have a drop-in new patient, your PVA will look deceivingly good. Therefore, always compare this particular computation with the other statistics and computations.

If all other statistics are holding steady and your PVA is low or dropping, numerous factors may be coming into play. While this statistic will not specifically tell you where the problem may be, it may give you an early "heads up" to a brewing problem. If you have a low or dropping PVA, you should look to the following causes:

- *Flawed new patient procedures.* Examine carefully your new patient procedures. Are you performing a proper consultation and examination? Are you using the new patient transition statements so that the patient understands your procedures?
- *Ineffective case review.* Is your report to the patient well conceived and well delivered and does it address the four questions the patient needs answered? Did you look for roadblocks or misunderstandings?
- *Inappropriate technique and adjusting room manners and mannerisms.* Do your adjustments hurt? Are you getting clinical results?
- *Inadequate attention to the patient.* Are you addressing the patient's concerns or talking about your interests? Are you listening to your patient?
- *Inconvenient office hours.* Can patients make convenient appointments for their adjustments or are they having to repeatedly take off work because of your office hours? Are patients waiting more than 10 minutes for their adjustments on a regular basis?
- *Mishandled appointments.* Are multiple appointment programs being properly utilized? Missed appointments recalled and made up on a consistent basis?
- *Ineffective patient education system.* Do patients understand the true promise of a chiropractic lifestyle?

♦ *Insufficient patient monitoring.* Are you reexamining and re-consulting with your patients, and keeping them up-to-date on their progress and need for future care?

♦ *Failure to continually coach patients.* Are you taking time to answer their questions and are you consistently educating them on a visit by visit basis?

These and many more activities will impact heavily on your patient visit average. But before you can understand how much influence each activity is having, you must quantify their effects. Watching your PVA is an excellent way to take the pulse of your practice over the long term.

Collection Percentage

The collection percentage is a reflection of the procedures, policies, and the staff's effectiveness in collecting for services that have been rendered. It is also a reflection of the effectiveness of the insurance and billing department. Although the monthly percentage will vary, a longer-term view (quarterly) will provide an adequate impression of the office collections. Whenever a quarterly collection percentage drops below 95 percent, it is time for concern. Immediate attention should be given to the persons responsible for the collection of the practice's funds, as well as the policies and procedures that will impact the approach necessary to ensure success in this area.

$$\textit{Formula: Collection Percentage} = \frac{\text{Collections in \$}}{\text{Services in \$}}$$

A low collection percentage (less than 95 percent) can indicate several dangerous problems that must be caught and addressed immediately. Once a collection problem begins, the likelihood of turning it around with any individual patient is difficult and potentially destructive to the doctor-patient relationship.

A well-designed, clearly communicated, and effectively administered collection policy is the first prerequisite for high-collection percentages. The second is a staff person who has no personal problems with enforcing the program. Anytime the collection percentage drops, even for a few weeks, you must immediately recognize it, and make an effort to determine why.

Following are a typical areas to investigate:

- *Poorly designed financial policy.* Is your financial policy well designed, appropriate for the majority of your patients and their financial/insurance situation?
- *Financial policy under-addressed with patients.* Is the financial policy being reviewed with the patient, appropriate arrangements being made, and is a commitment from the patient obtained?
- *Insurance issues.* Is there a problem with your insurance department? Are filings being made according to your policies and guidelines? Are you using appropriate insurance coding?
- *Inconsistent financial policy.* Are you, the doctor, meddling with financial arrangements that are being made or have been made?
- *Undermining the CA's job.* Are you escorting the patient out the door, preventing the front desk CA from collecting?

Failed Appointment Percentage

The failed appointment percentage reflects the percentage of patients who were scheduled but failed to appear within 15 minutes of their appointed time. This computation is derived from the number of failed appointments divided by the number of scheduled appointments.

Formula: Failed Appointment Percentage = $\dfrac{\text{\# Failed Appointments}}{\text{\# Scheduled Appointments}}$

This calculation is extremely important in that it reflects on both the doctor's and the staff's ability to impress upon the patient the importance of the care. An unacceptable failed appointment percentage (over 5 percent) usually denotes a lack of patient education, patient motivation, or a lack of respect for the doctor, the practice, and the profession.

Like the PVA, this calculation gives a vivid snapshot of the practice as a whole. Whenever the failed appointment percentage rises above 8 to 10 percent, red lights and bell should start to go off. The practice management team must begin to investigate every other category of the practice to determine the cause. Remember, from time to time you will find an individual patient who will chronically miss their appointments, but when missed appointments become routine in your practice, it is time to act.

- *Inadequate wellness care communication with patients.* Look carefully at your new patient procedures as well as to the case review for insight into why the patient may not understand the importance of maintaining their schedule of care. It is important in this area that the doctor obtains an unpressured commitment from the patient for following through with care. If the patient feels that they are being coerced or pressured into accepting the doctor's recommendations, they will often comply at first, then begin the pattern of missing appointments.

- *Inconvenient office hours.* Are the office hours convenient for the majority of your patients? If not, patients will make an effort to receive care while symptomatic, but will discontinue when free of pain and don't wish to be inconvenienced.

- *Need for reexamination and review.* Patients may become discouraged with lack of clinical progress or have progressed past symptomatic care and do not understand the objectives of correction and wellness care. Check your case review and recommendation presentation to the patient. Reexamine the patients, and review their progress and further health goals.

Income Loss Because of Failed Appointments

This often-dramatic figure shows how much income is lost because of failed appointments. Whether or not the rescheduled failed appointment percentage is high, a failed appointment still represents financial losses for the practice because the time reserved for the failed appointment was not available for other patients.

Formula:	Income Loss Because of Failed Appointments	=	# Failed Appointments	X	Average Income per Visit

This calculation is kept only for informational and motivational purposes. During the course of the day it is often easy for both you and your staff to adopt the attitude that, "Mrs. Jones missed another appointment. She'll probably call later; that's just how she is."

But when these missed appointments are converted to (and viewed as lost) dollars, they suddenly become urgent and real. Charging for missed appointments, however, is seldom the answer—unless you want the patient out of your practice and your hair. More times than not, charging for missed appointments will only serve to alienate a patient who may already be disillusioned with your practice. To prevent other patients from picking up these bad habits, you must find out why the patient missed and correct this situation. Always remember that a missed appointment is a symptom, not the underlying problem. Calculating the income lost because of failed appointments can make the symptom seem much more acute, and serve as a motivator for the doctor and staff to take a good look at their procedures and policies.

Map Dropout Percentage

This percentage is a vital indicator, giving immediate feedback as to the effectiveness of the entire office procedures. It will especially demonstrate the educational and recommendational aspects of your patient management procedures. A high or rising dropout percentage should be cause for immediate concern and close evaluation of the reasons surrounding each individual patient dropout.

$$\text{Formula: Map Dropout Percentage} = \frac{\text{\# of Dropouts}}{\text{\# of New Patients}}$$

In more advanced practices that utilize the multiple appointments scheduling procedure, this percentage will give immediate feedback as to the effectiveness of all the procedures in the office. This calculation will reflect directly on all of the activities and procedures discussed in the patient visit average and failed appointment sections. Conversely, the multiple appointment procedure will impact the patient visit average when properly administered.

Average Income per Visit

The average income per patient visit represents the actual dollar amount that each patient visit represents to the office on each individual visit. Too low of an average per visit income could represent a collections problem; too high may be detrimental to patient referrals, compliance, and longevity.

$$\text{Formula: Average Income per Visit} = \frac{\text{Collections in \$}}{\text{Patient Visits in \$}}$$

Average Income per Case

The average income per case or case average represents, on average, how much income (collections) can be expected from each new patient who enters the office. In other words, the case average is a financial valuation of each new patient.

$$\text{Formula: Average Income per Case} = \frac{\text{Collections in \$}}{\text{New Patients in \$}}$$

Such a valuation is critical to understand when determining the cost of attracting a new patient through various means. As an example, if a Yellow Pages ad costs $500 per month, but brings in five or six new patients each month at an average income per case of $1,000, it may be a procedure you may not want to drop if times get tight. However, if it only brings two new patients per month into a practice with a 50 percent overhead, you may be losing money on this procedure. In either case, this statistic provides valuable insight into the return on many of your marketing efforts.

The average income per case is an excellent means to quantify the financial appropriateness of many procedures. Remember, this calculation is a function of both collections and new patients. Always look at this section and make your subsequent practice decisions in reference to the health of both of these individual numbers.

A Final Thought

The chiropractic profession is the best hope for the continued upward evolution of humanity. Understood and properly applied, chiropractic represents a tremendous opportunity for every man, woman, and child to contribute to the full realization of global human potential. As the human race continues to evolve, environmental stresses will interfere as they always have, frustrating humankind's evolution to higher levels of understanding, decision making, and adaptation to ever-changing environmental forces.

Our existence today is proof of such victories. Likewise, as we learn to successfully deal with our environmental, physical, and cultural challenges, we, too, will pass our new knowledge on to our descendants. Much of this knowledge will be at the innate and cellular level, more at the conscious environmental and cultural level. Either way, only by successfully managing today's struggles will we be able to genetically encode and transfer this knowledge to our offspring. The operative word, of course, is "successfully." If such exotic viruses as we are seeing today kill us before we learn (as a species) to successfully deal with them, our children and their children will have to fight this same battle until someone figures it out or until our species perishes.

By building upon our ancestors' victories, we now have the ability to do everything from battle the once deadly influenza virus to putting men into outer space. Unfortunately, we are still living at the mercy of new and mutating viruses, and we are still polluting our internal and external environments. At some point, someone in this, or a future generation will develop the means to fight off the HIV or the Ebola virus, and humankind will learn to live in harmony with their world on a physical and spiritual level. These people will survive, they will multiply, and they will genetically pass this information on to their children and their children's children. However, to be successful, these individuals must be able to assemble all of their innate forces to win these ongoing wars. They must function at the high mental and physical levels that will give them this extraordinary adaptability.

Only those whose internal intelligence can call upon all of their current resources will acclimatize, thrive, and pass on these special adaptive abilities. Only those who live in a high state of subluxation-free wellness will possess these special abilities. This is the impact of chiropractic's greatest contribution to humanity. This is, indeed, natural selection at its best.

To be able to touch many lives and to makes such contributions, chiropractors must wear many hats. We must become teachers, motivators, and mentors. We must learn and develop new ways to educate and enlighten our patients so that we will ultimately change our collective consciousness as it relates to health and wellness. Consequently, that is why we must design policies and install procedures that not only allow and encourage members of our global society to avail themselves of our care, but to do so on a level that will allow us to effect species-altering changes. We must touch as many individuals and families as the hours in the day will allow. We must develop practices that attract the young and the old, the rich and the poor, and the vital and the frail. In short, we must build effective and efficient practices on the understanding of our immense vision of chiropractic and its promise for humanity.

This book is my contribution to helping chiropractors create these types of practices as the vehicles that will allow them to serve the masses, develop subluxation-free individuals, and assist humankind to adapt and advance through the generations that follow. It will take you from analyzing your physical office to developing patients who "get" chiropractic. At the same time, the policies, procedures, and concepts taught in this book will allow individual doctors to reduce the stress of practice and realize their personal dreams, goals, and the opportunity to experience the wonderful fulfilling life that chiropractic has to offer.

Enjoy reading this book again, study it, understand it, and employ its systems, policies, and procedures. Together, one patient at a time, from initial intensive care to lifelong wellness we can ensure the future of humankind. We can get the big idea.

About the Author

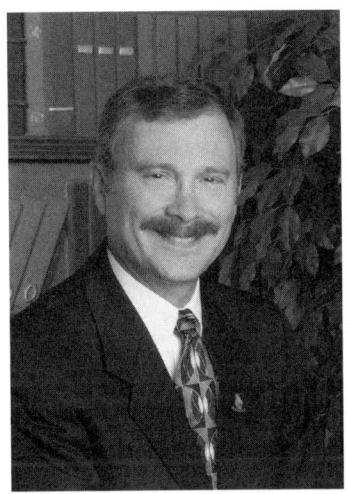

Dr. Mike Meyer is a chiropractic practitioner and president of Professional Practice Resources, Inc., a regional practice management consulting firm. He is a 1975 graduate of Palmer College of Chiropractic, Davenport, Iowa. He has been in active practice for nearly 30 years with as many as four multiple doctor offices serving both the metropolitan and rural areas of northern Indiana. Dr. Meyer has been active in state and alumni activities, serving as president of the Palmer College of Chiropractic International Alumni Association. In 1992, he was named a fellow in the Palmer Academy of Chiropractic. In 2003, he was named a "Distinguished Fellow" of the International Chiropractor's Association, and he has served as a senior consultant to the Palmer Institute for Professional Success. A frequent lecturer, Dr. Meyer was instrumental in developing the Palmer Institute's "Transition to Success" program for senior students and recent graduates.

Along with his wife Carol, who has served as the manager of their practices since 1976, Dr. Meyer has worked to help other doctors develop successful, proactive, profitable practices that provide high quality and professional chiropractic care to their communities. Dr. Meyer has established and quantified innovative procedures and systems to lower the procedural and financial barriers that limit the ability of patients to access chiropractic offices. Doing so, has resulted in such procedures as the modified cash practice, objective-based recommendations, and sustained referral techniques. Through this book, he hopes to share with other doctors the techniques, procedures, and successes that enabled him to bring chiropractic to large segments of his community.

Index

A

Achievements, quantifying 313-324
   average income per case 324
   average income per visit 323-324
   collection percentage 320-321
   failed appointment percentage 321-322
   failed appointments, income loss from 322-323
   MAP dropout percentage 323
   office statistics, categories of 314-317
   patient visit average 318-320
Adjusting rooms 20-21
Altered nerve transmission 207-213
American Red Cross 40
Appointment arrangements 214-224
Appointment book system 89-90
Appointment scheduling 76-77
Appointments, declined, procedure for 80-81
Appointments, missed 81-84, 246-251
   making up of 249-254
      benefits of making up 250-254
Audio brochure 38-39
Authorization to care for injured employee form 127

B

Beliefs, examining chiropractic 2

Braggard's Sign 170
Brochures 37, 67
   audio 38-39
Built to Last: Successful Habits of Visionary Companies 9

C

CA, phantom 59-67
Carnegie, Andrew 304
Case management and recommendations 225
Case management plans (CMP) 76-77
Case review cover, sample 200
Cervical distraction 169
Chiropractic assistant 18
   phantom 60-61
Chiropractic patients, creating lifelong 183-232
   adjustments, making patient's first momentous 230-231
   appointment arrangements 214-224
   case report, the 193-204
      case review 197-199
      case review, script of 199-201
      description of 196-197
      four questions 201-204
   financial review 214-224
   MAP procedure 224-230
      initial series 227
      scheduling tips 228-230
      second series 227-228

recommendations 186-188
  condition-based care 186-188
  for initial intensive care 186
  grade I 189
recommendations, clinical 193-195
recommendations, grade-based 186-188
  grade I 188-189
  grade II 189-191
  grade III 191-193
Chrysler Corporation 304, 305
Collins, James C. 9
Communicaton, effective 304-305
Complimentary consultation and exam certificates 39, 300-301. *See also* referral certificate
Condition-based care
  corrective care 187
  making recommendations for 188
  patient triage and objective-based recommendations 188
  relief care 187
  spinal stabilization 188
Confidence, in technique and in oneself 305
Corrective care 187
Courtroom testimony 93-94
CPT code 75

D

Directive for disbursement form 115, 220
Disc involvement 206
Distinctive benefit statement 288
Doctor-patient relationship and informed consent form 148
Dreams, importance of 4-5
Dreams, of perfect practice 5-9, 306

E

Education, continuing 309-310
Environmental link 284

Established patient update form
  back 262
  front 261
Examination/x-ray/consultation room 21-22
Expert witness 93-94

F

Family health history form 276, 278
Fee schedule, establishment of 27-30
Financial policies, creating 97-131
  insurance reporting procedures 117-123
  options for the cash patient 99-101
    arrangements for 100
    collection procedures for 100-101
  options for the insured patient 101-106
    coverage, verification of 101-102
    financial review 107-110
    first day fees, collection of 105-106
    first day's fees, discussion of 102-105
    insurance/co-payment, determination of 107-110
  patient/payment type, determination of 98
  personal injury cases 110-116
    financial options for 114, 116-123
  Workers Compensation 123-130
    dismissal letter 128-130
    pre-injury status dilemma 128
    written authorization 126
Financial review 214-224
  cash patient, determining payments for 217
  cash patient, possible arrangements for 221-224
  financial options, giving the patient 217-221

◆ Index ◆

introduction of 213
major medical coverage, determining payments for 215-217
modified cash procedure 214
First visit, systems for 133-182
   adjustment, first-visit 184-186
      post-adjustment release 184
   adjustments, problems with first-visit 181
   concerns, anticipating new patient's 134-141
   consultation 157-164
      first impressions of the doctor 163
      new patient consultation worksheet 157-163
   doctor-patient relationship developing 156-161
      initial consultation 153-156
      pre-consultation 156-157
      risk management 156-157
      transition statements 152-153
   examination 164-172
      examination process 167-170
      pre-examination 166-167
   first day fees, successfully collecting 179
   first impressions, shaping 148-150
      hospitality 151-152
   insurance coverage, procedure to verify 155-157
   new patient information 151-152
      informed consent form 153-157
      patient payment options gorm 153
      personal and historical information 152
   patients, booking 138-141
   releasing the new patient 176-177
      dismissal, the 178
   second appointment, scheduling 180-185
      releasing the new patient 180-185
      spouse at report 180-185
   x-raying the new patient 172-173
      post-exam/pre x-ray statement 175-176
Foramina compression test 169
Four questions 202
Four vertebra diagram 205
Frame of reference 284
Front desk/reception area 18

G

Gaenslen's 170
George's Cerebral-Vascular Test 169
Goldthwait 170

I

Iacocca, Lee 304, 305
ICDA diagnostic code numbers 35, 75
Inactive patient
   managing returning 258-263
   recalling 85-89
Informed consent form 143, 149, 260
Insurance co-payment worksheet 216
Insurance coverage, procedure to verify 155-157
Insurance reporting procedures 91-92, 117-123
Insurance verification worksheet 102, 103, 151, 152

K

Kemp's 170

L

Lewin's punch test 170
Linder's test 170
Location, of your office 13-18
   long-term hapiness 306-308

M

MAP 228, 323. *See also* Multiple appointment program

331

Map scheduling calendar 226
Master-mind alliance 308-309
Maximum cervical compression 169
Mentor, finding a 308-309
Missed appointment log 82, 248
Multiple appointment program 96, 224, 228, 236
   introduction of 213
Muscle splinting (spasm) 207

N

Nerve impingement 206
New patient consultation worksheet 158
New patient information form
  back 146
  front 145
New patient information slip 139
Newsletters 39
Notice to insurance carrier 118

O

Objectives of care 210
Office, your, designing for success 13-43
  buying versus leasing 19
  community, becoming known in 35-42
    audio brochure 38-39
    brochures 37
    business announcement 40
    business cards 38
    chamber of commerce 35, 36
    church groups 35
    civic groups 35, 36
    complimentary consultation and examination certificate 39
    CPR and first aid instructor 40
    intramural sports 36
    letterhead 38
    neighbors 37
    newsletters 39
    public speaking 37
    thank-you notes 39
    volunteer organizations 35
    Yellow Pages 40-42
  decorating 20-23
    adjusting rooms 22-23
    examination/x-ray/consultation room 24-45
    front desk/reception area 20-21
    office, doctor's private 25-45
    patient education center 25
  equipment 23-25
    leasing or purchasing 24-25
    office equipment 25
    professional supplies 25
    x-ray machine 24
  expansion, physical, opportunities for 19
  fee schedule, establishment of 27-30
    cash-based 28
    insurance-based 29
  floor planning 20-23
    adjusting rooms 22-23
    examination/x-ray/consultation room 24-45
    front desk/reception area 20-21
    office, doctor's private 25-45
    patient education center 25
  forms 26-27
    business cards 26
    computerized scheduling 26
    computers and software 26
    patient account-keeping system 26
    patient forms 26
  layout 20-23
    adjusting rooms 22-23
    examination/x-ray/consultation room 24-45
    front desk/reception area 20-21
    office, doctor's private 25-45
    patient education center 25

location, how to find best 13-18
location, importance of 13-18
office hours 30-32
office systems 32-34
   clipboard and numbered room system 33
   ICDA codes 35
   patient information (PI) card 33
   statements of financial policies 34
Options for care 209

P

Palmer, B.J. 30
Palmer "Triangle of Care" 184
Patient agreement form 109
Patient agreement/cash form 222
Patient case review form
   back 125
   front 124
Patient consultation worksheet 72, 157, 297
Patient education center 23
Patient empowerment statement 285
Patient financial options form 147
Patient information (PI) card 18, 32, 33, 34, 69-73, 84, 89, 91, 92, 183, 193, 215, 225, 228, 229, 246, 257
   back 71
   front 70
Patient insurance response letter 122
Patient referrals, generating new 265-302
   complimentary consultation and exam certificates 299-301
   consultation, introductory telephone 291-294
      procedure, built on the referral request 292
      procedure, referral request 293
      procedures, implementation 293
      program concept 291-292
   from your healthcare classes 273-275
      complimentary examinations 274
   prospective patient phone call 295-299
   referral atmosphere, developing a 266-267
      advertising 267
      off the street 268
      referrals 267
   referral, reluctant 294-295
   referral request procedure 279-290
   referral strategies, consciously implementing 268-272
      conditions, creating that allow for 271-272
      law of obligation 268-270
   referrals, doubling sources of 273
   through families 275-279
Patient types
   cancelled appointment, can't reschedule 256-257
   leaves office without appointment 258
   nonprogrammed new 257-258
   uncontrollable 254-256
   vacation 257
   will call 256
Patients, keeping educated 233-264
   appointment reminder procedure 245-246
   control, importance of maintaining 254-258
   forbid missed appointments 246-251
      missed appointments, making up of 249-254
      staff responsibility in 247
   patient recall, importance of
   recall and recapture procedure 251-254

patients, managing returning
  inactive 258-263
patients, processing of returning
  inactive 260-263
status, determination of patient
  259
reevaluation procedure 234-243
  comparative report 241-243
  consultative update 237
  implementation of 236
  reexamination 240-241
wellness, patient, involving family
  243-245
Peale, Norman Vincent 10
PI card. *See* Patient Information Card
Porras, Jerry I. 9
Practice of your dreams, creating 5-9,
  306
Progress evaluation form (consultation)
  238
Progress evaluation form (examination)
  239
Prospective patient log 296
Prospective patient phone call 295-
  299

R

Reevaluation procedure 234-243
Referral certificate 300. *See also*
  Complimentary consultation and
  exam certificates
Referral request procedure 279-290
Relief care 187
Rhomberg's 170

S

Sample forms
  Authorization to Care for Injured
    Employee 127
  Directive for Disbursement 115,
    220

Established Patient Update
  back 262
  front 261
Family Health History 276
Informed Consent 149
Insurance Co-Payment Worksheet
  216
Insurance Verification Worksheet
  103
Missed Appointment Log 82, 248
New Patient Consultation
  Worksheet 158
New Patient Information
  back 146
  front 145
New Patient Information Slip 139
Notice to Insurance Carrier 118
Objectives of Care 210
Options for Care 209
Patient Agreement 109
Patient Agreement/Cash 222
Patient Case Review Form
  back 125
  front 124
Patient Financial Options 147
Patient Information (PI) Card
  back 71
  front 70
Progress Evaluation (consultation)
  238
Progress Evaluation (examination)
  239
Prospective Patient Log 296
Referral Certificate 300
Service Slip 74
Staff Meeting Agenda 58
Statement for Doctor's Report 120
Statistics Worksheet 315
Subluxation Examination 168
Sample letters
  Patient Insurance Response Letter
    122

Index

Workers Comp Release Letter 130
Workers Compensation Welcome Letter 129
Seminars, attending 309-310
Service slip 73-75, 74
Shoulder depression 169
Signage 16
SLR 170
Soto-Hall's test 170
Spinal stabilization 188
Staff, developing a stong and effective 45-64
  appearances, importance of 59-62
    call forwarding 60
    "phantom" chiropractic assistant 60-61
    signal-calling 60
    smart-ring 60
  coaching 59
    communications, daily 59
    staff meetings, weekly 60-61
  leading and motivating staff 63
  preparations of a successful employer 47-49
    employee handbook 50-57
    job description 47-48
    operations manual 48
  recruiting 51-57
    advertising the position and accepting resumes 51, 51-52
    hiring and integrating 51, 56-57
    interview, initial 53
    interview, second 55-62
    interviewing and testing 51
    references, checking 54-55
Staff meeting agenda form 58
Staff meetings, weekly 60-61
Statement for doctor's report form 120
Statements of financial policies 34
Statistics. *See* Achievements, quantifying
Statistics worksheet 315

Subluxation effects 203
Subluxation examination form 168
Symptoms 206
Systems, developing 65-96
  brochures 67-69
  case management plans (CMP) 75-77
    patient benefits 75-77
  charting 90-95
    changes, monitoring patient 93
    insurance reporting 91-92
    note-taking 91
    patient management during corrective care 94-95
    progress tracking 92
    testimony, courtroom 93-94
  communication 67-69
  inactive patient, recalling 85-89
    contact guidelines 88
    script for 87
  missed appointments 81-84
    script for 83
  multiple appointment programs (MAP) 76-77
    patient benefits 76-77
  patient information cards 69-73
  policies and procedures 65
  procedure for the declined appointment 80-81
  procedures for reappointing current patients 78-80
    script for 79
  scheduling 89-90
    appointment book system 89-90
  service slip 73-75
  special tactics 65
  unscheduled patient, contacting 84-85

T

Tangible accelerator 287
Toe and heel walk 170

Trendelenburg's 170

U
Un-narrative report 123

V
Valsalva's maneuver 169
Values, importance of personal 2-4
Values, system of 9-10
Vertebral subluxation complex 184, 205

W
What can I do? 212
Workers Comp release letter 130
Workers Compensation 123-130
   dismissal letter 128-130
   pre-injury status dilemma 128
   written authorization 126
Workers Compensation welcome letter 129

X
X-ray 137, 165, 172, 173, 183, 198, 204, 260
   equipment 22
      buying used 24
   new patient 153

Y
Yellow Pages 14, 40-42, 41, 42, 268, 280, 324

Give the Gift of
7 Solutions for Building Your Proactive Chiropractic Practice
to Your Friends and Colleagues

CHECK YOUR LEADING BOOKSTORE OR ORDER HERE

❑ **YES**, I want _____ copies of *7 Solutions for Building Your Proactive Chiropractic Practice* at $49.95 each, plus $4.95 shipping per book (Indiana residents please add $3.00 sales tax per book). Canadian orders must be accompanied by a postal money order in U.S. funds. Allow 15 days for delivery.

❑ **YES**, I am interested in having Michael S. Meyer, D.C., speak or give a seminar to my company, association, school, or organization. Please send information.

My check or money order for $_____ is enclosed.
Please charge my: ❑ Visa ❑ MasterCard
❑ Discover ❑ American Express

Name _____

Organization _____

Address _____

City/State/Zip _____

Phone_____ E-mail _____

Card # _____

Exp. Date_____ Signature _____

Please make your check payable and return to:
Professional Practice Resources, Inc.
2609 Greenleaf Boulevard • Elkhart, IN 46514.

Call your credit card order to: _____
Fax: 574-264-1471

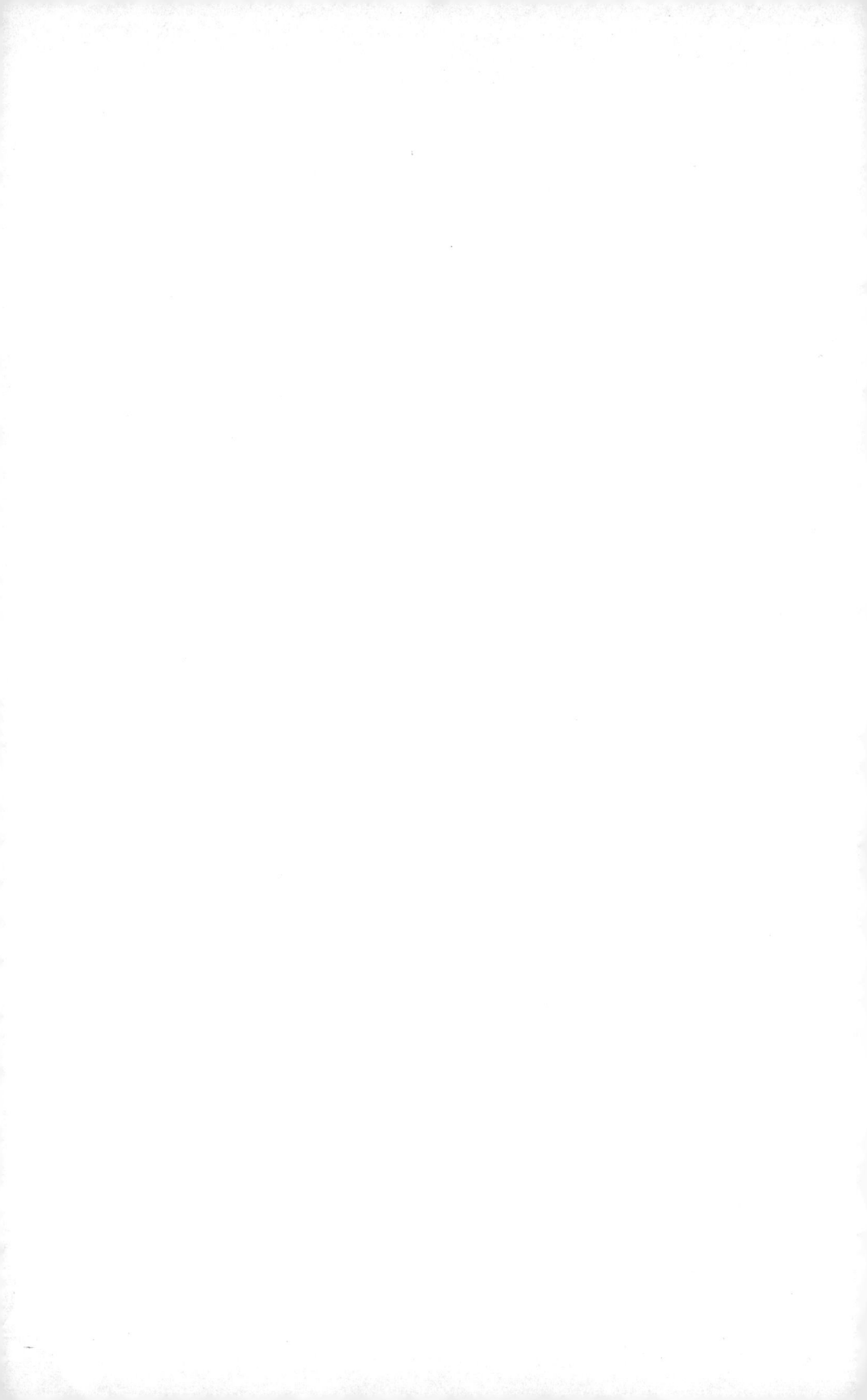